THE MANAGEMENT OF PET OBESITY

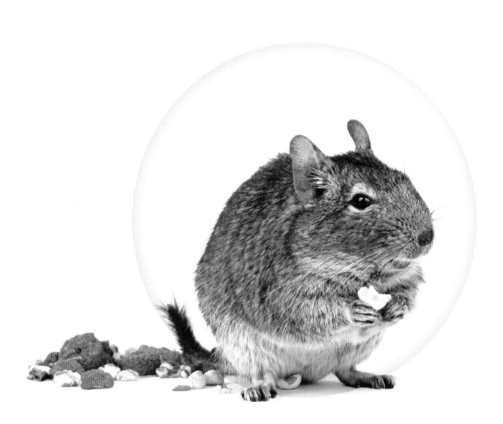

VICTORIA BOWES   HELEN COLEMAN

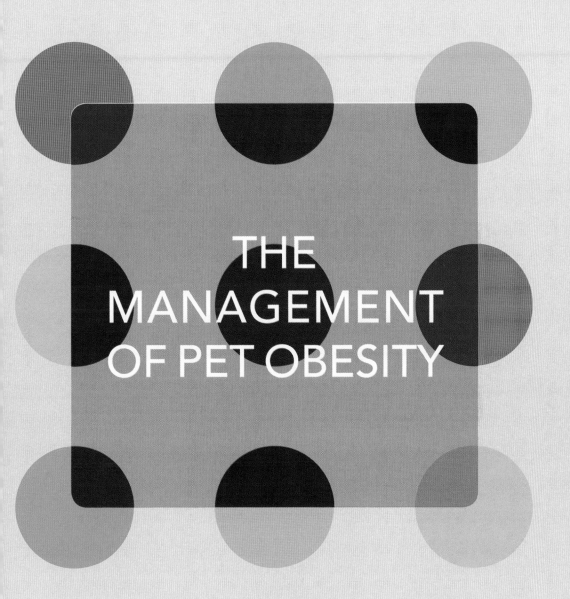

THE
MANAGEMENT
OF PET OBESITY

⭕ **5m** Publishing

Published by
5M Publishing Ltd,
Benchmark House,
8 Smithy Wood Drive,
Sheffield, S35 1QN, UK
Tel: +44 (0) 1234 81 81 80
www.5mpublishing.com

A Catalogue record for this book is available from the British Library

ISBN 9781912178346

Book design and layout by Alex Lazarou
Printed by Replika Press Pvt Ltd, India
Photos as credited in the text

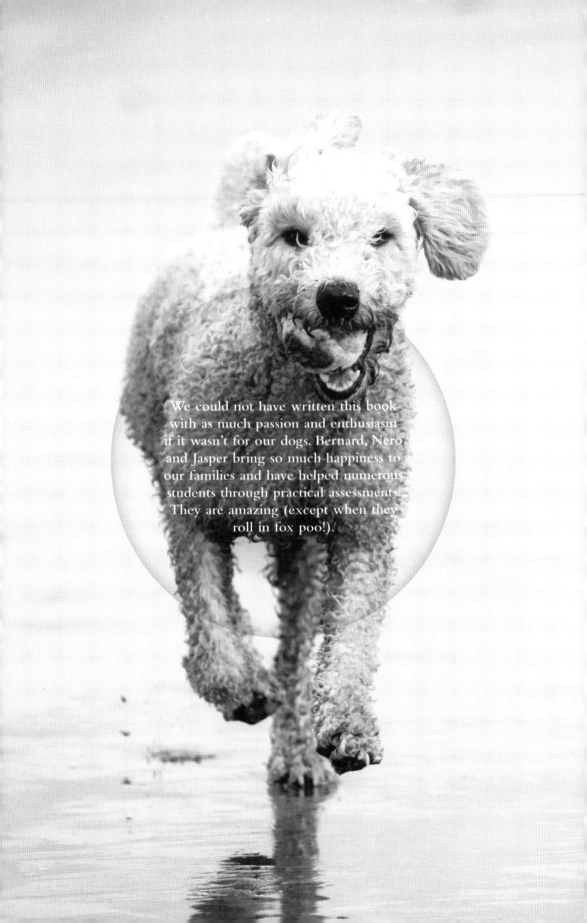

We could not have written this book with as much passion and enthusiasm if it wasn't for our dogs. Bernard, Nero and Jasper bring so much happiness to our families and have helped numerous students through practical assessments. They are amazing (except when they roll in fox poo!).

CONTENTS

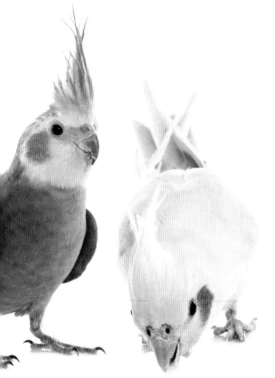

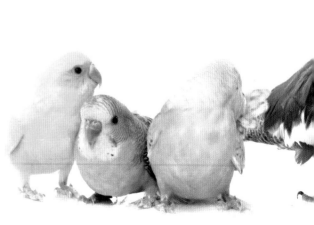

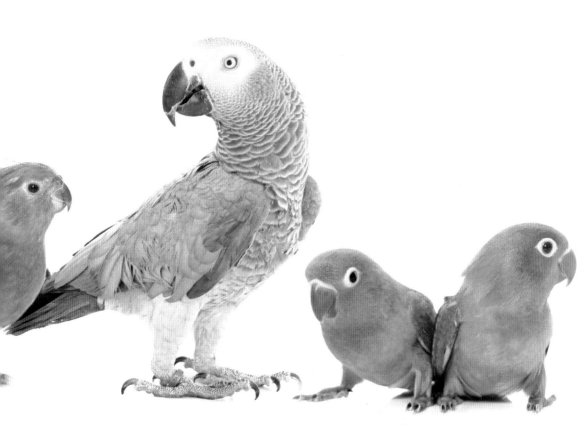

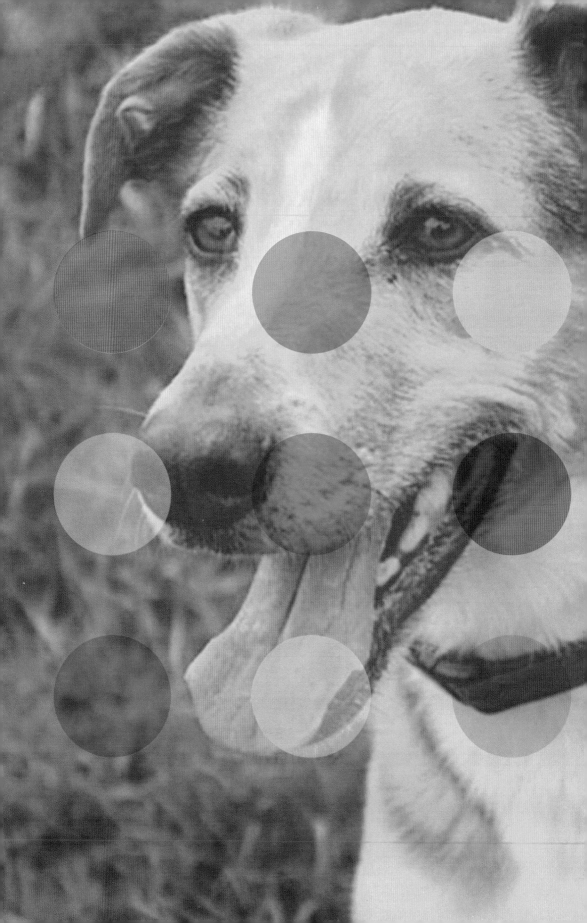

01
INTRODUCTION

PEOPLE LOVE PETS; they have become an ingrained part of human life providing companionship, emotional support, security, and can have a positive impact on human health and well-being. The humanization of pets is a reflection of the significance pets play in human lives and that they are very much part of the family. Many owners show their affection by 'treating' the animal and are often not aware of the calorific impact when feeding treats in addition to the daily recommended food allowance for the species, taking into account the breed, age or activity level. Many owners want to provide the very best for their pet are aware that nutrition is an important factor in promoting pet health. It is an owners responsibility to provide correct nutrition under the Animal Welfare Act 2006, but it can be difficult to make good nutritional choices when heavily influenced by clever marketing and advertising strategies. (The Act applies to England and Wales though secondary legislation is devolved. Scotland has the Animal Health and Welfare [Scotland] Act 2006 and Northern Ireland has the Welfare of Animals Act [Northern Ireland] 2011.) There is a wealth of nutritional research present online and in published material for pet owners but this can be contradictory and in some cases outdated; causing confusion to owners, practitioners and veterinary professionals.

We live in an age where obesity in humans is becoming commonplace and this is reflected in its acceptance in animals too. The way humans live their lives has a vast impact on an animal's state of health. An increase in sedentary lives reduces activity for both the human and animal but the food type and amount is not always adjusted to reflect activity levels. Animals too need a balanced diet that contains the six essential nutrients for optimum health, but this is not easily monitored when fed a home-made diet or human food, as it is a popular choice for some dog owners to feed table scraps. Many people have to work long hours which means spending less time with their beloved pet and they will often feed their pet extra treats to make up for their absence. Animals will not recognize the link between human absence and treats, but may associate certain human behavioural patterns with food time. Many owners cannot recognize when their pet is overweight and in many cases it is deemed 'normal'; there are many health-related issues associated with an overweight dog and these can be just as serious as those issues often seen in underweight dogs. Both are a welfare issue. Bland et al. (2008) categorizes dog factors that contribute to obesity as genetic disposition, reproductive management and diet.

Veterinary practices have a responsibility to monitor the rise of obesity in their clients' pets. They should recognize the importance of weight management clinics and how this role can be given to veterinary nurses which, in turn, may increase job satisfaction. Veterinary nurses have a key role with clients; sometimes, clients will speak more openly with the veterinary nurse providing an excellent platform to promote healthy pet weight.

Unfortunately, pet food manufacturers do not make the interpretation of pet food labels transparent and as a result the typical pet owner does not know what they are feeding. Better education is needed to help owners make more educated decisions on which type of diet they feed, for example feeding a proprietary diet; which brand provides the best value for nutrition in comparison to the amount it costs, how to use recommended feeding guidelines and what is a rational amount of treats to give in any one day. Furthermore, an important message for pet owners is to recognize the importance of companionship, training and exercise and the role this plays in enriching their pets lives instead of substituting with food; which in the long term will have detrimental effects on their pet's health.

OBESITY CLASSIFIED

An animal can be classified as obese when the body weight exceeds 10–20% of the recommended weight (German, 2006) and is defined as an accumulation of excessive amounts of adipose tissue in the body. Obesity is becoming one of the most common nutritional disorders in companion animals, often the result of either excessive dietary intake or inadequate energy utilization, which 'causes a state of positive energy balance' (German, 2006).

GENERAL CLINICAL SIGNS OF OBESITY IN DOG AND CATS

- Slower body movement
- Lethargy
- Exercise intolerance
- Excessive fat palpable over ribcage
- Specifically, in cats, belly dragging on ground
- Inability to groom effectively
- Dyspnoea

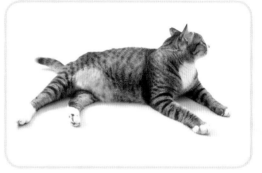

↳ An overweight cat.
Photo: Adobe Stock – silamime

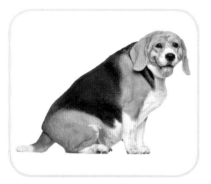

↳ An overweight dog.
Photo: Adobe Stock – Eric Isselée

EVOLUTION OF THE PROBLEM

The UK population is becoming more overweight with human obesity becoming an escalating global problem (German, 2006); 69% of American adults over the age of 20 are considered overweight, obese and extremely obese (National Institute of Health, 2011). Wedderburn (2015) reports that 51.5% of American adults will be obese by 2030, also predicting that the UK population is not too far behind.

This issue is reflected in the pet population and is a recognized welfare concern (German, 2006). Sandoe et al. (2014) identify regional variations in the levels of obesity in both humans and animals globally. Furthermore, the same report found that on a global scale, 22–44% of animals were considered obese.

Vets estimate that up to 45% of all pets they treat are overweight or obese (PFMA, 2015) and weight control is as relevant to pets as it is to humans (Mintel, 2011). The Pet Food Manufacturers Association (2015) indicates pet owners' awareness of pet obesity has improved by 30% since 2009, yet the PDSA's research estimates that 25% of dogs seen at its hospitals in the UK are overweight (Lund et al., 2006) suggesting that owners are failing to recognize and acknowledge signs of obesity in their own animals.

Companion animals are often regarded as valued family members (McNicholas, 2005) which signifies the strength of the human–animal bond; this is more prevalent in owners of obese cats. Owners often misinterpret cat-led interaction as a request for food even when their cats are not hungry; furthermore, if food is provided at such times, the cat soon learns that initiating contact results in a food reward (German, 2006).

In contrast, in humans and dogs, for whom eating is a social function, factors that are of importance for obesity recognition in pets include the duration the owner observes the dog eating (more likely to be longer in obese dogs); interest in pet nutrition; obesity of the owner; health consciousness of the owner (both for their pet and themselves) and lower income households (German, 2006).

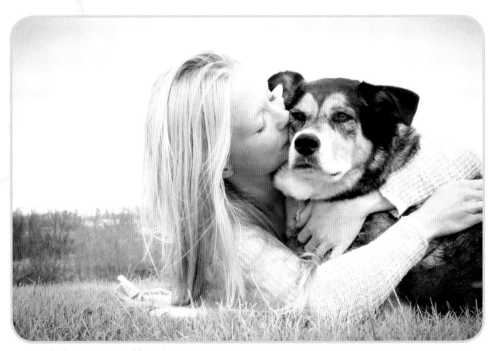

↘ The human–animal bond.
Photo: Adobe Stock – Christin Lola

A major problem in the prevention and treatment of canine obesity is compliance. Owners argue that they love their pet so much that they cannot deny it treats and, like cat owners, tend to interpret their dog's every need as a request for food. This in part could be due to a transfer of their own health and eating habits (Kienzle et al., 1998), thus disregarding warnings on possible health risks when it comes to portion size and normal feeding behaviours. Such behaviours are also evident in owners of pet birds as owners do not typically weigh food, instead topping up food bowls when they appear empty regardless of the amount consumed. It is important for owners to consider the daily energy expenditure when measuring feed rations; this is especially true for caged animals that have limited exercise opportunities, for example a pet bird who might be allowed free access for a couple of hours a day.

Owners commonly use human-based foods as treats and do not truly acknowledge the caloric impact on the animal. The PFMA reports a 28% increase over five years in cat and dog owners feeding pets table leftovers. The PFMA (2015) reports that these acts of apparent kindness are a leading cause of pet weight gain (78% for dogs).

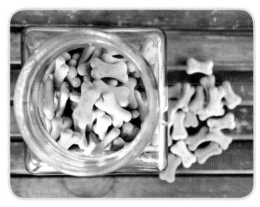

↪ Owners like to treat their pets.
Photo: Pixabay

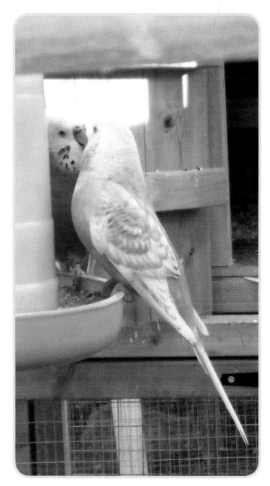

↪ Obesity in pet birds can occur if portion control is not monitored.
Photo: Darren Gibson

It's easy to want to express affection for a much-loved pet by rewarding them with treats, however 'titbits' should generally mean smaller main meals to compensate the caloric intake. PFMA (2015) findings show that nearly half (48%) of pet owners are treating pets more than twice a day. Guilt feeding is a common issue to compensate for failing to provide sufficient time, attention, exercise and companionship due to fast-paced, demanding lifestyles.

Advertising is becoming more targeted thus encouraging the feeding of high-fat, high-salt diets and treats. Two in three (68%) pet owners admit to not following professional guidelines (PFMA, 2015) when deciding portion size, and with 30% taking a cavalier approach relying purely on instinct.

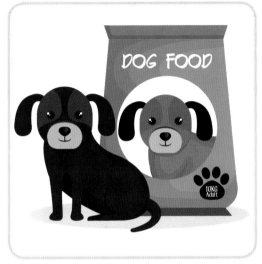

↘ Breed-specific advertising.
Photo: Adobe Stock – Gstudio Group

PRIMARY CAUSES OF PET OBESITY

Owners are responsible for the food the pet primarily consumes but other factors such as endocrine pathology and recovery from illness which could alter the metabolic and physical state should be considered. Neutering is an important risk factor for obesity in all species. Furthermore, many vets and most owners appear to treat this as an unavoidable association; perhaps it would help both groups to know that neutering can reduce energy expenditure by up to a third so it is imperative that the veterinary nurse educates owners when they have their pets neutered. Many recognized pet food manufacturers now offer specific nutritionally balanced diets to meet the needs of neutered pets.

Other predisposing factors can contribute to a change in feeding behaviour which can lead to decreased activity without a corresponding decrease in energy intake (German, 2006). Furthermore, gender itself is also a predisposing factor in indoor, middle-aged and apartment-dwelling cats (German, 2006). Also, specific canine breed factors can be linked, for example, the Labrador retriever appears to be more prone to developing obesity (Raffan, 2014). A shift from a working gundog often to a popular household pet has fuelled the obesity problem in this breed, however a breed predisposition suggests that genetics are also important in the genesis of obesity in certain breeds and ages which has prompted further opportunities for specific diet-related foods (Mintel, 2011).

MANAGEMENT

The PDSA (2014) reports that approximately 30% of the entire UK dog population of around 1.95 million dogs is overweight (Dog Nutrition, 2014). Others have suggested the prevalence exceeds that figure, rising to approximately 50% in dogs and cats between 5 and 10 years old (Lund et al., 2005).

One of the major issues is owner compliance and failure to recognize that their animal is overweight and to take responsibility for the situation. Nursing clinics can be a valuable source of education to allow owners to talk openly to the veterinary nurse about the importance of dietary management and obesity-related issues without the fear of being judged by a veterinary surgeon.

Weight management clinics enable the practitioner to closely monitor obesity on a one-to-one basis with the owner and track weight loss using graphical data. It can be useful to get the owner involved, thus taking responsibility for the situation and the impact on the animal using body condition scoring tools. Photographic evidence can be very helpful for a visual comparison. Education on dietary and exercise management, plus education on interpreting pet food labels can contribute to an organized weight loss programme. Industry professionals can play a vital role in the education of owners on how to calculate daily feed amounts by following recommended feeding guidelines on the food packet in order to meet the desired target weight.

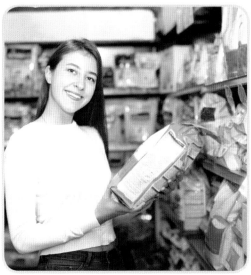

↘ Education can help pet owners make more confident decisions.
Photo: Adobe Stock – JackF

7

The PFMA (2015) found that only one in three (37%) pet owners know how to check their pet's weight, leading to misconception of the overall body condition. Rabbit owners in particular may not appreciate what is a normal or ideal body weight (Meredith, 2012) because there is currently no validated body condition scoring for rabbits (Cardinali et al., 2008), as for other species. Body condition scoring can be measured against a recognized scoring system produced by most recognized pet food manufacturers, however if at any stage it becomes evident that it is not a diet or owner-based issue then it needs to be referred to the relevant veterinary surgeon.

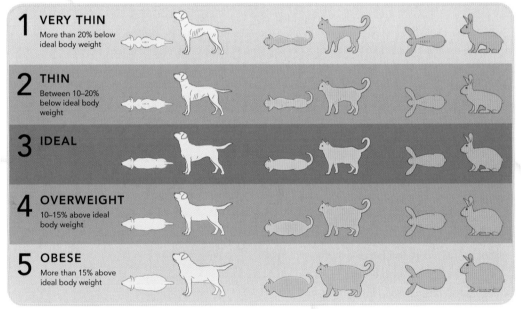

Body condition scoring of dog, cat and rabbit.
Photo: Artist: Jorgen McLeman

OBESITY-RELATED PROBLEMS

Excess weight can result in increased wear on the joints which may result in the early onset or worsening of osteoarthritis and skeletal disorders, thus compromising the quality and enjoyment of life due to impaired locomotion. Dental, gastrointestinal disease and behavioural problems (Meredith, 2012) may also be associated with inadequate diet regimes although respiratory- and cardiac-related problems can result in increased predisposition to other metabolic diseases leading to a shorter lifespan.

SUMMARY

Pet obesity is on the rise and will continue to increase unless substantial education of owners is common practice as obesity in companion animals is a serious medical concern (German, 2006). Literature plays an important role with waiting rooms and information boards being the ideal location for pet obesity displays. Many pet owners are open to support and would welcome guidance which can be provided by industry professionals to promote the health and well-being of their animals (McNicholas, 2005). 'Prevention is better than a cure' and the pet industry must take some responsibility in actively educating owners on the weight management of their pets.

HANDY HINT
HOW TO MANAGE OUTDOOR CATS AND MULTIPLE HOUSEHOLDS:

- Tags that read 'do not feed'
- Inform neighbours
- Reduce food availability at home
- Separation feeding
- Move away from ad lib feeding to time and amount restricted.

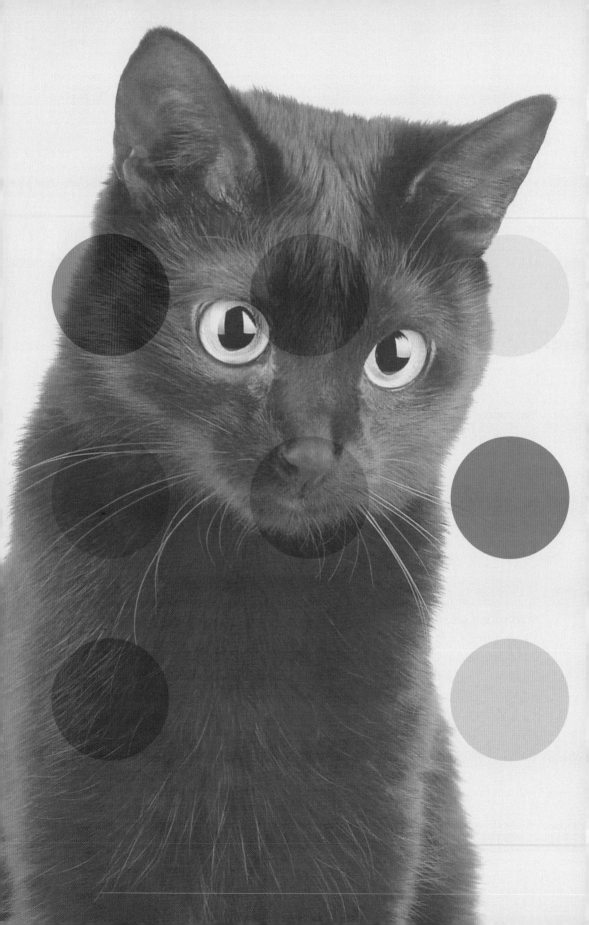

02
THE NUTRIENT REVOLUTION

A BALANCED DIET contains all the essential nutrients to ensure the correct functioning of the body and maintenance of the animal's health. A complete diet is important for energy, growth, repair and reproduction.

Some nutrients are essential and therefore must be provided in the diet as they cannot be synthesized by the body, or in specific disease states. Furthermore, nutrients can also be classified as non-essential, are produced by the body and therefore not an essential daily dietary requirement; but should be present within the diet.

Energy is obtained by eating food which provides nutrients to supply energy and gives the cells power to function. An animal cannot use all the energy supplied in food; some energy is used and lost in faeces, urine, gas and digestion of food.

Gross energy is the removal of faecal energy to become digestible energy. This works really well with simple monogastric animals such as pigs, dogs and humans. Digestible energy becomes metabolized energy when urine and gas is released. Gas losses from ruminants can be very high in methane. Metabolized energy becomes 'net' energy; this is the 'ready' energy source available for use. The body commonly uses it for maintenance functions and production of heat which can heavily affect energy use due to thermal regulation.

CALCULATING MAINTENANCE ENERGY REQUIREMENTS (MER)

The resting energy requirement (RER) needs to be calculated in order to obtain the MER. To calculate RER you need to know the body weight of the animal and to take into account energy expenditure and environment.

RER = 30 × body weight (kg) + 70 = resting energy in kilocalories (Kcal)

MER = RER × 1.4 (cats)
MER = RER × 2 (dogs)

TABLE 2.1

DAILY ENERGY REQUIREMENTS FOR HEALTHY CATS AND DOGS

1 hour light work	MER x 1.1
1 full day's light work	MER x 1.5
Gestation post 3 weeks	MER x 1.1–1.3
Birth to 3 months	MER x 2.0
Sub-freezing temperatures	MER x 1.7
Tropical heat	MER x 2.5

ADDITIONAL ENERGY NEEDS FOR ENVIRONMENTAL CHANGES

→ **ACTIVITY**

Calculate the total extra energy requirement for the following questions:

1. Calculate the change in caloric requirements for an 8-kg West Highland terrier after completing one hour of light work.
2. Calculate the change in caloric requirements for a 35-kg German shepherd in sub-freezing temperatures.
3. Calculate the change in caloric requirements for a 3-kg cat in tropical heat conditions.

CASE STUDY

FLOSS

An entire, female 4-year-old working Collie, weighing 20 kg; works on the farm daily with her owner and two other dogs. She lives outdoors in a kennel which has an external heat source and protection from the elements.

Floss has a daily requirement of 2010 Kcal per day. The farmer followed the daily feeding guidelines on the feed packet to ensure the calorie needs were met. Floss has a lean body condition score and would be graded at 2 on the 5-point BSC scale.

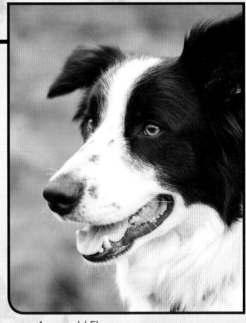

↳ 4-year-old Floss.
Photo: Pixabay

DRY MATTER ANALYSIS

The dry matter analysis can be calculated to determine the nutrient value of food. The proportion of ingredients such as fat, protein or carbohydrates in food varies; the moisture content can impact on the quality and amount of the nutrients.

Using the food label as a comparison of nutrients can lead to inaccuracy and is potentially misleading. Comparing the dry matter analysis is a more accurate method of determining the nutrient content.

To be able to compare different types of moist and dry food you first need to remove the water content. Then you will be able to compare the percentage of food content.

Water content is provided on a typical food packet. If the water content is not listed then you must assume it is 10%; it is required by law to list anything above 10%.

The following calculations are used to find out the dry matter analysis.

Weight of food (g) - moisture content % = dry matter %

Then the percentage of the nutrient/% dry matter × 100 = actual % of nutrient

This answer gives the correct amount of nutrient in the food per 100 grammes.

Example:

100 g weight of food
10% moisture content
20% fat

100 g -10 (%) = 90% dry matter

20 (% fat)/90 (dry matter) × 100 = 22.2% of fat.

THE NUTRIENT REVOLUTION

All animals need energy for homeostasis; the amount of energy required depends on age, sex, size, activity level, environmental conditions and physiological status. See Chapter 7 on life-stage diets.

There are *six* main nutrients, which can be divided into energy-producing nutrients:

○ Protein
○ Fat
○ Carbohydrates

and non-energy-producing:

○ Water
○ Vitamins
○ Minerals.

We will explore these, and the role they play in an animal's metabolism, in turn.

Protein is an important food component needed for growth and repair and plays a vital role in the production of antibodies. Antibodies help to protect the animal and build immunity and strengthen muscle extension and contraction. The requirement for protein depends on the species, age, life stage, activity level and health status.

Proteins are divided into 23 amino acids. Some are essential and have to be present in the diet and fed on a regular basis because animals cannot produce them. Examples include lysine, tryptophan and valine.

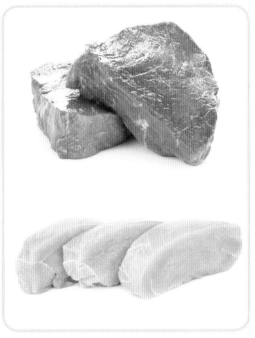

↳ Meat is a primary protein source.
Photo: Adobe Stock – karandaev; Evgeny

There are ten essential amino acids in the dog and 11 in the cat. Cats and ferrets are known as obligate carnivores and *must* have animal protein in their diet – this extra essential amino acid is known as *taurine*. Non–essential amino acids can be made by the body from other amino acids.

Sources of protein essentially include meat, fish and dairy products but can also be found in pulses, legumes and nuts. Proteins are made up of a combination of different amino acids. These are converted into carbon, nitrogen and oxygen atoms that join together in a 'condensation reaction'. During this process they lose a molecules of water and form peptide bonds to make up peptide chains. Some of these are classed as complex proteins and the different amino acids form into polypeptide chains.

The biological value can be measured by the quality of protein and how digestible it is by the body. If the biological value is low then digestibility is poor meaning the animal needs to consume a higher amount of protein to compensate for the low quality. On the other hand, if the protein quality is high, less is needed to meet the daily nutritional requirement of the animal.

TABLE 2.2
THE BIOLOGICAL VALUE OF COMMON PET FOOD INGREDIENTS

FOOD	BIOLOGICAL VALUE
Egg	100%
Fish meal	92%
Milk	92%
Liver	79%
Beef	78%
Soybean meal	67%
Meat and bone meal	50%
Whole wheat	48%
Whole corn	45%

DEFICIENCY

Deficiency occurs when an animal is not provided the appropriate amounts of nutrition or if a medical illness inhibits the animal's ability to absorb nutrients effectively.

Clinical signs of nutritional deficiency
- Poor growth, skin lesions
- Weight loss, poor appetite
- Impaired immune function, healing and repair
- Loss of coat condition (rough and dull)
- Hypoproteinaemia

Taurine (cats only)
As obligate carnivores, cats require a meat only-based diet due to the need for taurine which is found only in animal proteins such as chicken and duck.

- Seen in cats fed dog or vegetarian food
- Feline central retinal degeneration, impaired immune function, poor reproduction, abnormalities in kittens and can also cause a serious heart condition termed dilated cardiomyopathy.

CASE STUDY

SMOKEY

Smokey is an 18-month, male, neutered domestic shorthaired cat. His owners had decided to feed the cat dog food to stop the dog eating cat food, as it was gaining weight. The cat was fed on dog food for approximately three months and was presented to the vet in a collapsed condition. Upon investigation, it was diagnosed by the veterinary surgeon that Smokey was suffering from dilated cardiomyopathy. The condition of the cat proved fatal due to a lack of taurine in its diet which has led to a taurine deficiency. The taurine deficiency was due to the dog food not being supplemented and not containing sufficient amounts of taurine to meet the requirements for Smokey.

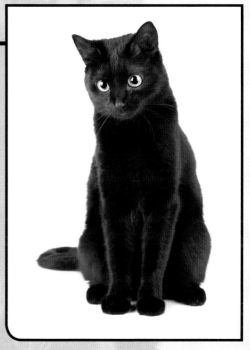

⤷ Smokey the cat.
Photo: Adobe Stock – Ekaterina Garyuk

EXCESS

Animal practitioners and guardians have a responsibility to provide sufficient amounts of nutrition to ensure good animal health. It is commonplace to supplement a diet with additional food sources, however, if fed in too large quantities excess can build, resulting in toxicity.

○ Can be used for energy or stored as adipose tissue
○ Ammonia removed from protein is converted to urea by the liver and excreted via the kidneys

○ Excess amounts of urea can overwork the kidneys and can cause damage; this is especially relevant in older cats.

→ **ACTIVITY**

For an animal species you know or work with:

1. List five of the roles of proteins and explain their importance in the maintenance of health in the animal's body.

2. Identify five sources of protein that can be fed to an animal.

FATS

Fats are also known as oils and lipids; these are the most efficient nutrients for providing energy to the animal, providing 2.25 times more energy than protein or carbohydrates. Fats provide essential fatty acids and are essential for the body to store fat-soluble vitamins A, D, E and K. Fat is also notorious for improving the palatability of food.

Fats have several functions in the animal's body. They are needed to:

○ Store energy; when excess energy from fat is not used it is stored as a fat cell for future use to provide energy

○ Transport vitamins; vitamins A, D, E and K are fat soluble meaning they are absorbed into the lymph (waste) fluid in the body. They are then transported via carrier proteins into the bloodstream. Excess vitamins can be stored in the liver or as fat cells for future use

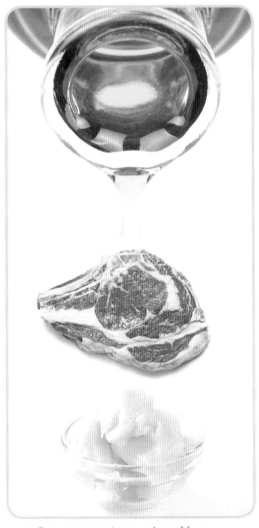

↳ Fats can come in a number of forms.
Photo: Adobe Stock – paketesama; Pavlo Kucherov; Viktor

○ Assist with the protection of body organs by providing padding to the outside of the organs

○ Assist insulating the body by providing a fat layer underneath the skin; this aids in heat retention and production.

Some fats are essential to the animal's well-being and are known as essential fatty acids (EFAs). Most species can synthesize linolenic acid from linoleic acid which is required by most animals. Another essential fatty acid is arachidonic acid, which is only found in animal fats and is essential to the cat, as other species are able to synthesize this from linoleic acid found in the diet.

While some fats are necessary in the diet, excess can result in weight gain, thus obesity, steatorrhea and vitamin E deficiency. But too few EFAs can lead to a dull, scurfy coat, alopecia, skin lesions, impaired wound healing, anaemia, infertility and finally, at end stages, fatty liver degeneration.

The most common form of dietary fat are triglycerides, classified as saturated, mostly found in animal fats, for example butter and lard; unsaturated, commonly known as olive and linseed oil; and polyunsaturated, such as sunflower oil.

Fats may be:

○ Saturated: a saturated fat is solid at room temperature; each carbon atom is bonded to two hydrogen atoms. Saturated fat is found in meat and dairy products but also nuts like coconuts and cashew

○ Monounsaturated: an unsaturated fat is liquid at room temperature; in monounsaturated fat, two of the carbon atoms are only bonded to one hydrogen atom and instead form a 'double bond' to each other. Monounsaturated fat is found in seeds like olives, flax and sesame

○ Polyunsaturated: which have many double bonds, and include the omega 3 and 6 fatty acids. Polyunsaturated fat is found in fish, cereal and seeds such as sunflower.

➔ **ACTIVITY**

Choose a species of animal and consider the foods that are most likely to provide them with good sources of fat.

How might this differ for another species such as a dog, hamster or finch?

CARBOHYDRATES

Carbohydrates are a very reliable source of energy and fibre. Carbohydrates can be found in fruit, vegetables, potatoes, rice and cereals. Carbohydrates can be considered as non-essential food components for dogs and cats and are commonly used in animal feed as a more cost-effective form of energy. Carbohydrates are often used to bulk out food to give more density and have a low caloric value. Carbohydrates have several functions in the animal body. They are key for storage and transportation of energy and assist with important physiological processes such as the immune system. When in its fibre form, it can assist with digestion and excretion.

Carbohydrates can be divided into soluble (digestible); sugars and starches and insoluble (indigestible); and cellulose.

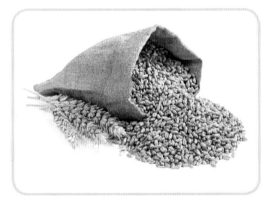

↘ A form of carbohydrate.
Photo: Adobe Stock – Timmary

Simple carbohydrates or sugars usually taste sweet, can be digested quickly and enter the bloodstream rapidly. They include glucose, fructose and galactose (monosaccharides) and lactose, sucrose and maltose (disaccharides). Sugars are found in a range of foods, such as fructose in fruit and lactose in milk.

Some useful definitions

○ Polymer: a long molecule containing a very large number of smaller molecules
○ Monomer: these are repeating units that make up the polymers.

Disaccharides are the combination of two simple sugars. One common form is sucrose – this is the sugar you put in your tea. In its natural form, it cannot be absorbed by the body. It undergoes chemical breakdown so it can be split into smaller, absorbable components.

Oligosaccharides are composed of 3–10 bonded monosaccharides. For example, amylase is a glucose polymer. This can be formed as a repeating monosaccharide or a mixture.

Polysaccharides can be thousands to millions of units long. They are present in all plants and animals. Common polysaccharides include glycogen and starch.

Carbohydrate deficiency

Carbohydrates are effectively classed as non-essential; however, a lack may result in other nutrients being used as an energy source. If not enough fibre is consumed in the diet, this can result in constipation.

Carbohydrate excess

Fibre increases faecal bulk (diarrhoea) and reduced absorption of other nutrients.

→ ACTIVITY

1. What are good sources of protein for:

   a) cats
   b) rabbits
   c) finches

2. What are the three main types of fat?

   a)
   b)
   c)

3. What is the difference between simple and complex carbohydrates?

WATER

Approximately 70% of the mammalian body is made up of water and it is the most important nutrient needed for homeostasis, cellular reactions and respiration. A daily intake of fresh water is required to replace obligate water loss from the body. Intake can be derived from drinking water and from food (70% water content in moist food and 10% in dry food) and is needed to maintain normal electrolyte balance.

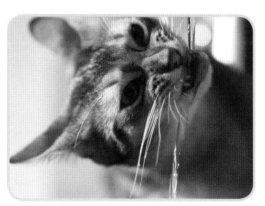

↘ Fresh water should always be available.
Photo: Adobe Stock – goodween123

Water is essential to aid in thermoregulation and lubrication of body tissues. A 15% loss of water would lead to death. Water loss occurs naturally through urination, defecation, sweat and milk production. Dogs pant to reduce body heat, which cause evaporation of water from the tongue. Cats sweat from their paws – you can see this when they walk on a smooth, reflective surface.

VITAMINS

Most manufactured dog and cat food that is produced on a commercial scale is fortified with vitamins that tend to exceed the recommended minimum requirements. This is not necessarily an immediate cause for concern for the animal since the body will utilize what it requires or dispose of the excess when within safe limits. Dogs and cats have no specific requirement for additional vitamin C in the diet as they are able to synthesize this within the liver. Although there are some benefits to supplementation, vitamin C is an antioxidant with a natural affinity for free radicals. It is an absolute essential requirement to provide a vitamin C supplement in the diet for guinea pigs as they are not able to synthesize vitamin C within the body and a deficiency will result in scurvy. There are complete diets available on the pet market which meet the necessary vitamin C requirement although it is still recommended to supplement the diet of a guinea pig with a range of fruits and vegetables to add variety and enrich the diet. There are other ways to supplement, such as liquid drops that are added to water, although it is important to follow manufacturers' instructions and be aware to avoid presenting this form of supplement in a traditional drinking bottle as the aluminium spout will inactivate the vitamin C. Supplements should not exceed 10% of the total food intake.

Vitamins are involved in most essential body functions.
However, they are only needed in small amounts and are divided into:

- Fat-soluble vitamins
- Water-soluble vitamins.

Fat-soluble vitamins (A, D, E, K)

Fat-soluble vitamins need a safe amount of fat within the diet for their absorption and storage. They are not needed daily in the diet as they can be effectively stored and if offered in too large quantities, excess fat will be stored.

TABLE 2.3a

FAT-SOLUBLE VITAMINS

VITAMIN	SOURCE	FUNCTION	DEFICIENCY	EXCESS
A (Retinol)	• Fish oils • Egg • Liver • Kidney • Green vegetables • Carrots	Assists the visual pigments in the retina of the eye and assists with the growth of bone and teeth. It also maintains healthy skin and assists kidney function.	Can cause skin and eye lesions; results in poor growth and major reproductive problems.	Anorexia, weakness, pain, lameness, stiffness, bone hyperplasia. Can result in liver damage in dogs and cats.
D (Calciferol)	• Fish oils • Egg yolk • Milk • Can be synthesized by exposure to sunlight	Absorption of calcium and phosphorus from intestine and the maintenance of calcium levels. It is also very important for bone and teeth formation.	This usually is rare when a balanced diet is fed. When the calcium and phosphorus ratio is imbalanced it can cause rickets in young animals and in adults it can result in osteomalacia which is softening of the bone.	This can result in calcification (hardening) of soft tissue and certain organs. Also results in bone and teeth malformation especially in immature animals.
E (Tocopherol)	• Milk • Animal fat • Green vegetables • Cereal • Liver	This is a key antioxidant. It also prevents fat turning rancid. In synergy with selenium it protects the cell membrane.	In cats it can result in pansteatitis (yellow fat disease) due to being fed an excess of oily fish. In dogs it can result in muscular dystrophy and poor reproduction.	None
K Phyltoqui-none	• Green vegetables • Can be synthesized by intestinal bacteria • Can be destroyed by out-of-date feeds • Can also be destroyed by sunlight and certain types of food processing	This is very important for the normal function of blood clotting.	Increased haemorrhage and extended clotting times. Can also cause anaemia and hypoprothromb-inaemia.	None

Water-soluble vitamins (B group and C)

These cannot be stored in the body so must be provided daily in the diet or via supplements. Dogs and cats can produce vitamin C from glucose in the liver, but humans, primates and guinea pigs cannot. If the vitamins are provided in excess they are usually excreted in the urine.

TABLE 2.3b

WATER-SOLUBLE VITAMINS: B AND C GROUPS

VITAMIN	SOURCE	FUNCTION	DEFICIENCY
B1 (thiamin)	• Liver • Cereals • Dairy products • Yeast • Is very sensitive to excessive heat and will degrade.	Important for carbohydrate and protein metabolism.	Can result in poor growth in immature animals. Anorexia can be apparent, with neurological signs, leading to heart failure and then death.
B2 (riboflavin)	• Yeast • Milk • Liver • Kidney	Important for carbohydrate, fat and protein metabolism.	Can result in weight loss. Can cause poor growth in immature animals. Generalized weakness can be seen. Skin disorders can be seen.
B6 (peridoxin)	• Egg • Liver • Yeast • Fish • Cereals	Important for protein metabolism and growth in young animals.	Can cause anorexia. Anaemia can be viewed on blood profiles. Diarrhoea can be seen and poor growth in immature animals. Can result in irreversible kidney damage in cats.
B12 (cobalamin)	• Heart • Milk • Egg • Liver • Kidney • Excess can be stored in the body.	Important for blood cell production within the bone marrow.	Can cause anorexia, In immature animals it can result in poor growth. Its key function is being involved in blood cell production, so deficiency can result in anaemia and leucopaenia.
Pantothenic acid	• Egg yolk • Liver • Legumes • Yeast	Involved in fat and carbohydrate metabolism.	Very rare as present in most products which are included within animal feed.

VITAMIN	SOURCE	FUNCTION	DEFICIENCY
Niacin	• Fish • Liver • Dogs can convert tryptophan into niacin.	Involved in fat, protein and carbohydrate metabolism. It is extremely important for healthy oral and pharyngeal tissues.	Can result in black tongue. Oral ulceration resulting in drooling and severe halitosis. It is seen in dogs that are fed solely corn-based diets.
Biotin	• Various meat products • Liver • Milk • Yeast • Green leafy vegetables • Can be synthesized by intestinal bacteria.	Has a key role in gluconeogenesis mainly for the production of energy. It is important for growth of the immature animal. It also helps maintain a healthy skin.	Can result in dry, scurfy skin and alopecia. It can also result in hyperkeratosis causing a hardening of the skin.
Choline	Plant and animal material.	Involved in fat metabolism. It is also involved in the messenger functionality of the neuron.	Quite unlikely as it is commonly found in all animal and plant foods.
Folic acid	• Fish • Spinach • Yeast • Kidney • Liver • Legumes • Can be synthesized within the intestine.	Important for blood cell production within the bone marrow.	Quite rare due to intestinal bacteria synthesis.
C (ascorbic acid)	• Fruit (high in citrus) • Vegetables • Can be synthesized from glucose in dogs and cats. Increased when the animal is stressed and is increased in neonates. • Can be destroyed by excessive exposure to heat.	Important for the formation of bone with a role in osteoblast function. It is involved in the transport of iron. It supports and encourages active wound healing.	Can result in decreased appetite and poor growth in immature animals. Swellings can form around the joints, a generalized weakness can be seen and sometimes bleeding gums – this is scurvy.

Note: Excess is not usually seen as when not needed they are excreted in the urine.

MINERALS

Minerals can be classified into three major categories. Macrominerals are required in a gramme weight level per day; microminerals are required in a weight of mg per day and, finally, trace minerals, which are still unclear in their role. A balanced diet is necessary to provide the correct amount of minerals and can result in poor intestinal absorption if sufficient quantities of minerals are not provided. Trace minerals can be involved in various bodily functions.

TABLE 2.4
FUNCTIONS OF MINERALS IN THE ANIMAL'S BODY

MINERAL	FUNCTION
Chromium	This is required for the biochemical digestion of carbohydrates.
Cobalt	Component of vitamin B12.
Fluoride	This is important for teeth and bone development.
Molybdenum	This is important for various enzymatic functions.
Nickel	This maintains the functions of membranes.
Silicon	This is important for both bone and connective tissue growth and development.
Vanadium	This is important for reproduction and growth and is involved in fat metabolism.

TABLE 2.5
MACROMINERALS

MINERAL	SOURCE	FUNCTION	DEFICIENCY	EXCESS
Calcium	Bonemeal, milk, cheese.	Development of bone and teeth, nerve and muscle function, blood clotting.	Nutritional secondary hyperparathyroid-ism causing rickets or osteomalacia. Eclampsia at whelping (large) and mid lactation (toy) causing twitching and convulsions.	Skeletal problems in young, rapidly growing dogs, e.g. HD. Calcium oxalate crystalluria or uroliths in adults (cats).
Phosphorus	Bonemeal, milk.	Development of bone and teeth, utilization of energy.	Stiff, poor hair coat, weakness, inability to raise head, kidney failure in cats on high protein diet. Due to low potassium diet (cats) or excessive loss due to diarrhoea.	Rare, not known.
Potassium	Milk, meat (linked to protein intake).	Water balance, nerve and muscle action, protein synthesis.	Exhaustion, dry skin, hair loss, poor growth, fatigue.	Rare; thirst, high blood pressure (long-term).
Sodium	Common salts, milk, meat, eggs.	Nerve and muscle action, water balance.	Muscle weakness, depression, unlikely to be seen (poorly formulated struvite prevention diets).	Diarrhoea, struvite urolithiasis.
Chloride	Common salts.	Water balance.		
Magnesium	Cereals, bone, green vegetables.	Development of bone and teeth, energy metabolism, enzyme activation.		

TABLE 2.6
MICROMINERALS

MINERAL	SOURCE	FUNCTION	DEFICIENCY	EXCESS
Iron	Eggs, liver, green vegetables.	Forms part of haemoglobin, utilization of oxygen.	Anaemia, weakness, fatigue. Young fed inappropriate milk substitutes.	Weight loss, anorexia.
Iodine	Fish, shellfish, dairy produce.	Forms part of thyroid hormone.	Goitre, alopecia, weight loss, lethargy, drowsiness.	Similar to deficiency.
Copper	Meat, bones, fish.	Formation of bone and haemoglobin, melanin production.	Anaemia, bone disorders.	Anaemia, hepatitis (Bedlington terriers).
Manganese	Liver, kidney.	Component of connective tissue, enzyme function, fat and carbohydrate metabolism.	Degeneration of skeletal and cardiac muscles.	Death seen within hours to days due to pulmonary oedema (other species).
Selenium	Meat, offal.	Linked with vitamin E and can replace it to some degree.	Hair loss, skin thickening, poor growth, skin lesions.	Rare; vomiting, weight loss, anaemia, anorexia (coins), diarrhoea, may interfere with the absorption of iron and copper.
Zinc	Liver, fish, shellfish.	Helps in digestion and tissue maintenance, correct wound healing, healthy immune system.	Can cause growth problems.	Neurological clinical signs, e.g. ataxia.

CASE STUDY

BILLY

Billy, a 6-year-old severe macaw, was fed solely on a seed-based diet for many years without supplementation. Seed-based diets are high in protein and fat; digestion of these nutrients results in high levels of urea which causes damage to the kidneys during excretion. Parrots are known to select feed and will chose the most palatable seeds (usually sunflower seeds or peanuts), with the highest fat content. In the latter years, Billy started to present clinical signs of significant renal failure and was diagnosed by a veterinary surgeon. The extent of the damage proved fatal and was likely to be caused by hypovitaminosis A.

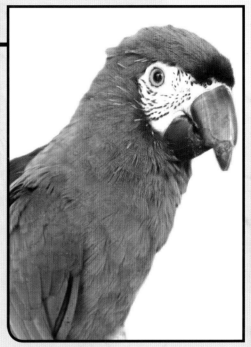

↘ Billy the parrot.
Photo: owner

ADDITIVES

Most formulated diets will have some form of food additive to enhance the nutritional value, palatability or visual appeal. An additive is essentially a substance that is intentionally added to perform a specific function; a good example would be sweeteners but other technological additives include preservatives, antioxidants, emulsifiers and acidity regulators.

Additives may also stimulate various sense organs which include flavours and colours and current thought processes lean towards a link between food aroma and palatability. A highly palatable food will in turn be more appealing if it has a strong aroma as this will stimulate the olfactory senses of the animal, although Phillips-Donaldson (2012) suggests that the aroma also has an effect on owner choice.

Added flavours are given to increase the palatability of food and to enhance the likelihood of consumption. Some artificial flavours are not natural and are added to increase acceptability of the food to the animal. Some foods have additional salt and fat added to them as it is known that these play a role in palatability, however, excess salt can affect the heart and too high fat content can lead to obesity.

In dogs and cats, it is thought that colours are added more for owner benefit than the animals', as colours and shapes make the food look more exciting to the owner and good marketing of pet foods, encourages the owner to purchase the food. Dogs and cats have a limited colour spectrum, yet this is different for avian species as parrots are highly selective of food items based on texture, size and colour.

Additional additives can include:

○ Anti-cracking agents: used to prevent food from clumping together
○ Emulsifiers: prevent fat and water separation
○ Mould inhibitor/antimicrobial: these are used as they prevent spoilage of the food
○ Antioxidants: these prevent fats from becoming rancid
○ Chemical preservative: used to enhance the shelf life of the food and to prevent the food from spoiling.

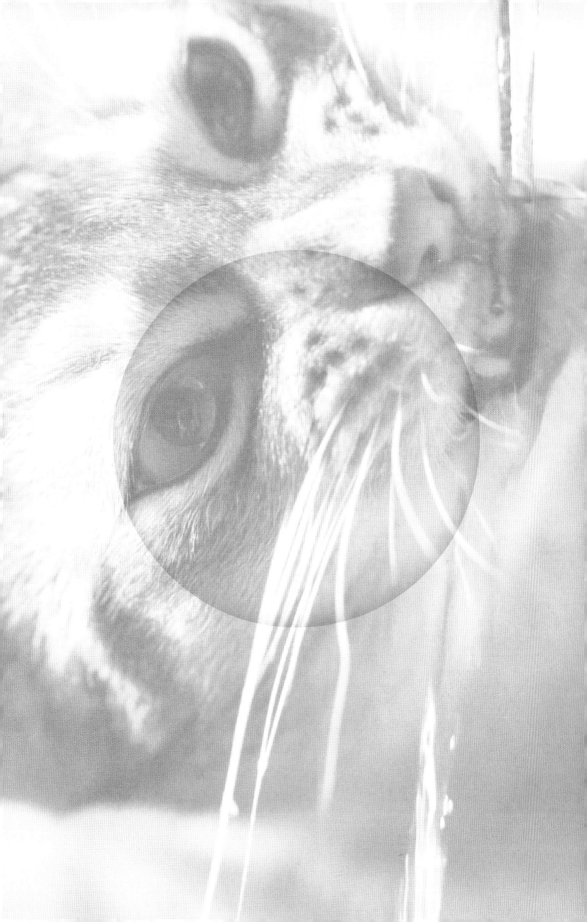

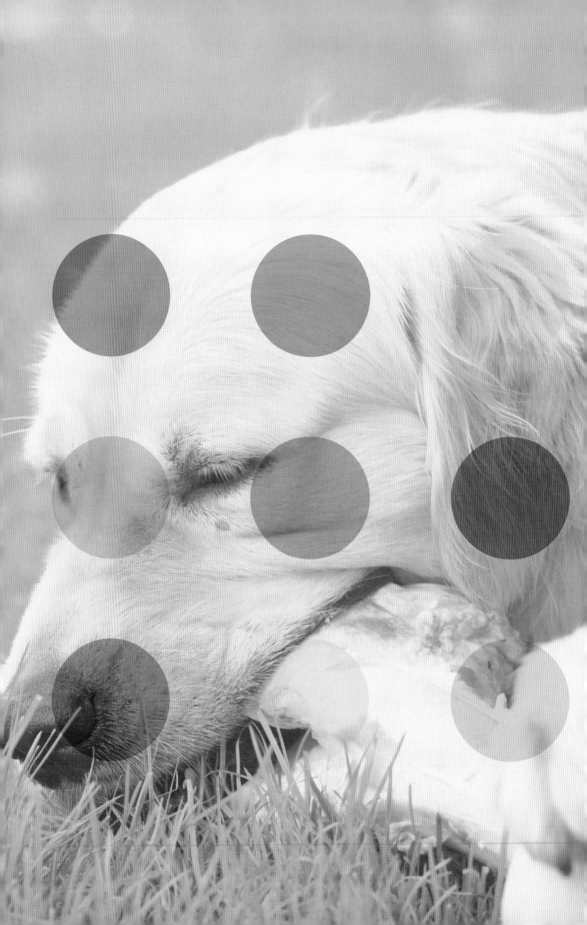

○ ○ ○

03
COMMON MISCONCEPTIONS OF FEEDING

○ ○ ○

THERE ARE A NUMBER of dilemmas pet guardians face when trying to make the right decision about what to feed to their pet. There are many myths surrounding the correct way to feed your pet. There is no right or wrong answer, but there are many considerations that need to be taken into account in order to ensure your pet receives a healthy and balanced diet.

Can I feed my dog table scraps?

Basically, there are connotations to feeding human food to dogs. In essence, the feeding of titbits potentially provides the dog with additional sugars, fats and salts which can lead to an unbalanced diet and potentially contribute to disease.

Is it safe to feed bones to my dog?

Many people choose to feed an evolutionary fresh diet which is reported to have health benefits of a healthy coat condition, promote good dental health and provide higher energy levels. There are

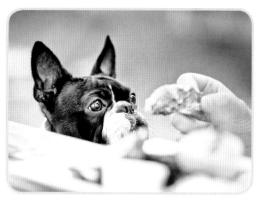

↘ Feeding table scraps.
Photo: Adobe Stock – Nailia Schwarz

CASE STUDY

ERIC

The owners took on a young, challenging Great Dane. Training was one of the first priorities and the dog trainer would only work with Eric on a natural diet. This was to ensure they were working on his base behaviour, without the influence of ingredients from a manufactured diet (we know what impact additives and colourants can have!). The raw diet of tripe started to have a positive impact, not only on behaviour, but his coat condition improved and his weight evened out too. The owners were so pleased with the results, they now feed all four of their dogs a raw diet. Buying in bulk is a more cost effective way of feeding this type of diet as they get through 10 lb of food per day.

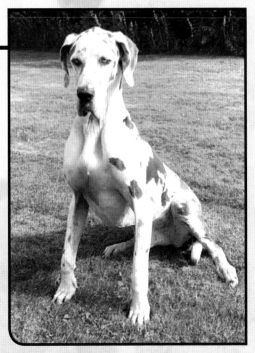

↘ Eric the Great Dane.
Photo: Natasha McCarty

concerns in the veterinary world associated with giving bones to their dog with regards to the risk of impaction. Never feed boiled bones as the cooking process softens and causes them to splinter which can harm the digestive tract. Poultry bones are also too soft and can cause the same problems as boiled bones.

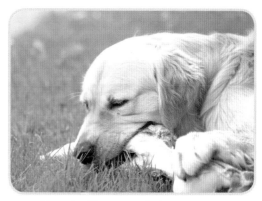

↳ Uncooked bones can help to promote good dental health.
Photo: Adobe Stock – Robert Emprechtinger

Can I feed dog food to my cat?

A canine diet does not contain a sufficient amount of taurine which in the long term can cause deficiency to the feline, leading to various medical conditions and potentially life-altering disease.

Can I feed rabbit food to my guinea pig?

Guinea pigs are classified as caviomorph which is a group of animals that, like humans, cannot synthesize vitamin C. Rabbit food is not supplemented with additional vitamin C to meet the needs of your guinea pig and if fed long term can lead to deficiency-related disease.

CASE STUDY

SNUFFLES

Snuffles, a guinea pig, lived with a rabbit called Thumper. The owner did not understand the importance of nutrition and fed them both on rabbit food. This resulted in the guinea pig developing a vitamin C deficiency, presenting with diarrhoea, poor condition, limited locomotion and weight loss. Snuffles was then administered a vitamin C supplement and changed to a complete balanced diet specifically formulated for guinea pigs. Regrettably, the health implications of the deficiency were too developed and resulted in Snuffles being put to sleep.

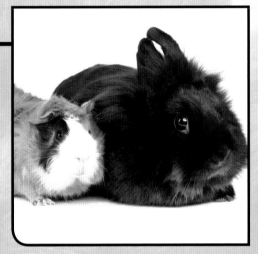

↳ Snuffles and Thumper.
Photo: Adobe Stock – Magalice

Can I feed live vertebrate animals to my reptile?

In the UK under various pieces of animal welfare legislation it is an offence to inflict pain or suffering to any vertebrate animal, therefore feeding a live rodent to a snake could result in injury to either party and can lead to prosecution.

I feed a home-made diet to my dog – is this safe?

Feeding a home-made diet has many benefits as you can control the quantity and quality of the ingredients, which is attractive to many pet guardians. Naturally, the better quality the ingredients, the more benefit to the animal. You must, however, ensure that you are meeting the nutritional requirements of the dog in order to offer a balanced diet, which can be challenging. A carefully calculated home-made diet will provide some security that you are meeting these needs which offering table scraps does not. Feeding a

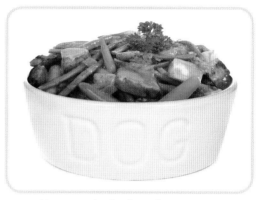

↳ Home-made diet for a dog.
Photo: Adobe Stock - adogslifephoto

proprietary diet is very convenient for pet owners and provides a safe and consistent diet providing manufacturers' guidelines are followed, but only when feeding guidelines are followed.

MODELS OF RAW FEEDING

Biologically Appropriate Raw Food is part of the raw feeding revolution that follows the concept of canines as omnivores. This is the diet of choice for some pet guardians due to its natural composition which resembles the diet of a domesticated dog. The composition of this diet generally comprises of meat, muscle meat, bones, organs, offal, fruits, vegetables and sometimes dairy. Supplements can be added depending on animal health and food availability. Veterinary advice should be sought before making dramatic changes to a raw-based diet.

Conversely, the prey model is based on the philosophy that dogs are true carnivores and they are offered muscle meat, meat, bones and offal. And not offered plant matter.

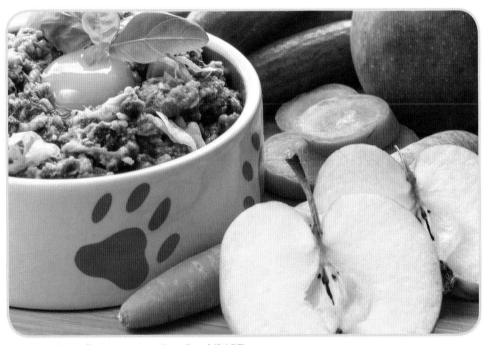

↳ Biologically Appropriate Raw Food (BARF).
Photo: Lilli

Let's start from the beginning. The first interaction most people have with a brand or type of food is usually with an advert or campaign. Marketing is very powerful and emotive but this does not necessarily demonstrate the quality of the diet advertised. Emotive pictorial stories used as part of an advertising campaign are designed to resonate with the emotional part of our brain. The company aims to draw in the consumer and resonate with the brand as opposed to the product itself. Brand loyalty is important to manufacturers. This is where owner education is essential in the selection of the product based upon the quality rather than fancy packaging. Understanding the food analysis is crucial to selecting the right food for your pet.

These definitions will go some way to helping you make some good choices:

○   Complementary suggests that the diet is not balanced and is in 'addition' to another ingredient/diet. You need to add a base food to make this complete.
○   Complete, as it suggests, contains all the necessary ingredients that the animal needs in that meal. You do not need to 'complement' the food with anything else, otherwise you run the risk of unbalancing the formulated diet.

○ Proprietary refers to a manufactured, branded food.
○ Meat flavour: does not have to contain the animal as stated.
○ Contains or with: only needs a minimum of 4% of that animal.

It is important that you understand food labelling when making decisions about what diet is best. Manufacturers use specific terminology which can be difficult to interpret if you do not know what to look for.

The following definitions will help you to make more informed decisions the next time you pick up a bag of pet food.

Fresh meat is an excellent source of protein and increases the palatability of food. Do not be fooled into thinking this is the equivalent to a nice piece of steak – this human-grade meat is essentially the viscera left behind. Fresh meat has a high water content and increases the mass of the food when initially added but water is removed during processing and the amount of meat in the final product is reduced.

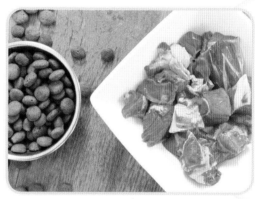

↘ Fresh meat used in pet food.
Photo: Monika Wisniewska

Dry meat meal is far more nutritionally dense than any other type of meat product. As the name suggests, the meat is dried and water extracted before it is added to the food base and the quality of the meat is retained.

Bone meal does not contain any specific animal product and although it is a good calcium and phosphorus supplement it can be linked to food intolerances, for example to chicken.

Animal derivatives are the lowest grade of meat and the animal of origin cannot be given as it can simply be a mixture of hair, skin, nail, bone or feather from any freshly slaughtered, warm-blooded animal. On the other hand, animal derivatives do potentially provide a mixture of protein sources. This can be particularly problematic for pets with food intolerances.

UNDERSTANDING FOOD ANALYSIS

For any animal practitioner or pet guardian, interpreting the labels on the packaging of pet food can be a challenge but it is important to understand the quality of food you serve to your pet. The ingredients listed are the guaranteed composition of food, usually expressed as a percentage. The golden rule of thumb is that ingredients are listed in order of quantity, with the highest content listed first. So, for example, if cereals are listed at the top of the food analysis label, the proprietary diet contains more cereal included than anything else.

Manufacturers will often use broad terms such as 'cereals' or 'meat and animal derivatives' for the simple reason that the quantities of ingredients may change from batch to batch. Cereals, for example, otherwise known as grains, can be categorized as wheat, maize, barley, oats and rice. Cereals provide an important source of energy, a proportion of protein and other nutrients including thiamine and niacin. These can often be in small quantities and listed separately, but when added together can make up a large proportion of the food. Cereals can be of varying quality; high-grade cereals include rice, oats and barley, however, grains such as sorghum are not high-grade as this ingredient is high in starch and is typically considered nutritionally poor. On the other hand, sorghum is gluten-free and can play an important role in foods provided to dogs with food intolerances. Alternative fibres such as beet pulp or rice bran are palatable fibre sources and can have additional beneficial effects on the health of the digestive tract and stool quality (De Godoy, Kerr and Fahey, 2013).

There is much debate around the use of cereals within dog food as they are generally low-grade ingredients and tend to be a cost-effective method to bulk out the food. Where most manufactured dog foods commonly include some form of carbohydrate, diets that contain this as their main ingredient should generally be avoided unless you can be certain of the type of cereal. Brown rice is a cereal favoured by many manufacturers as it is highly digestible, nutrient-dense and promotes good digestive health.

○   Ash is not an added ingredient but is reflected as a percentage on the pet food label. Manufacturers carry out a test in which they incinerate the food at high temperatures, burning off all the organic components such as carbohydrates, fats and proteins and leaving behind the minerals (hence, a pile of ash). It is important to be aware of the mineral content of food to avoid excess or deficiencies.

EXTRUDED PRODUCTS

Extrusion has been used in the pet industry for many years. Most of the available animal feeds have been manufactured using the extrusion process that involves the ingredients being mixed, sliced and heated under high pressure. This is then forced through a shape-making die to form a ribbon-type product which is then dried and turned into kibble.

The extrusion process is completed by cooking at a high temperature for a short duration; this process creates various chemical and physical changes to the mixture.

These changes can include:

○   Changes in nutritional quantities and quality, specifically vitamin loss
○   Starch can become gelatinized
○   Protein can become denatured.

A degree of nutrient loss is inevitable during the manufacturing process. On average dog and cat food contains approximately 30–40% starch, which when exposed to heat and moisture melts and binds the product together. After the extrusion process many kibble diets may have changes in glucose and so it is not reliable for diabetic animals.

BULKING AGENTS

Bulking agents are added to kibble to provide bulk or mass to a specific food, but it must be noted that although it increases the size of the food, it has limited nutritional value. It is usually cheap for manufacturers to buy, hence being added into food instead of providing the food full of pure meat/vegetable. One of the most common bulking agents is cereals. Bulking agents can be used in lower-priced weight-reducing diets as they are specifically designed to expand and make the animal feel fuller. Owners must be aware that some bulking agents used can be higher allergen responders. Owners of animals with wheat allergies must ensure they fully read the ingredients. If the term 'bulking agent' has been used, you cannot guarantee that wheat is not within the food.

TREATS

Treats are typically fed as a reward and the amount of treats given should be monitored across the day. When feeding or advising the owner about treats the following must be considered:

- Caloric impact: treats and their calories must be considered as part of an animal's daily recommended caloric intake. Whilst treating an animal is seen as a positive action by pet guardians, education on calorimetric maintenance must be considered.

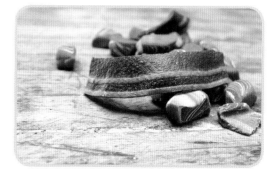
↳ Treats.
Photo: Adobe Stock – reezabrat

- Overfeeding: some pet guardians will choose to use the animal's main diet as part of the treating system. This is a particularly useful way of offering rewards as long as the daily amount of food is not exceeded.
- Fat, salt and sugar are included to make treats palatable and sensory-stimulating.
- Behaviour: most owners will use food as a reward to reinforce behaviour when training. High value food items are often chosen to keep the dogs interest. Owners must compensate by adjusting the daily ration of food to compensate for additional calories.

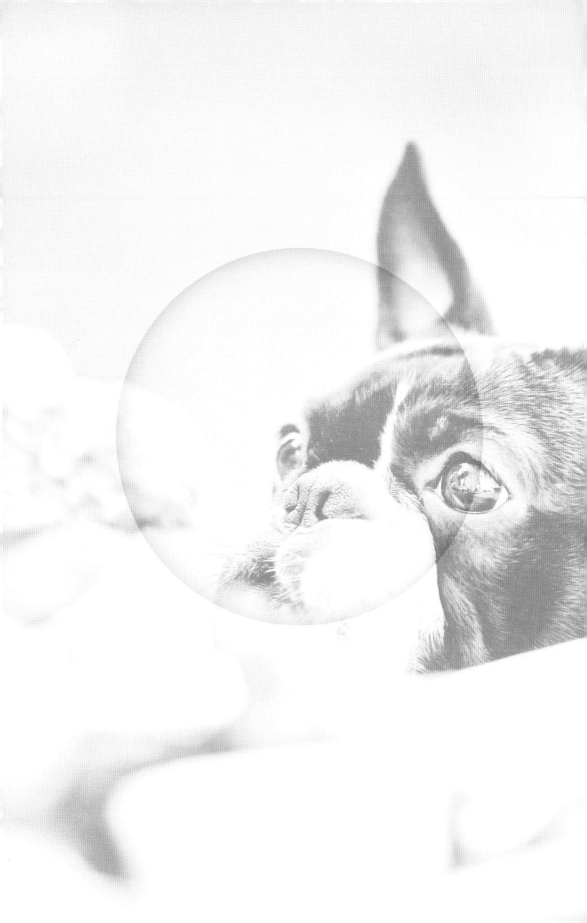

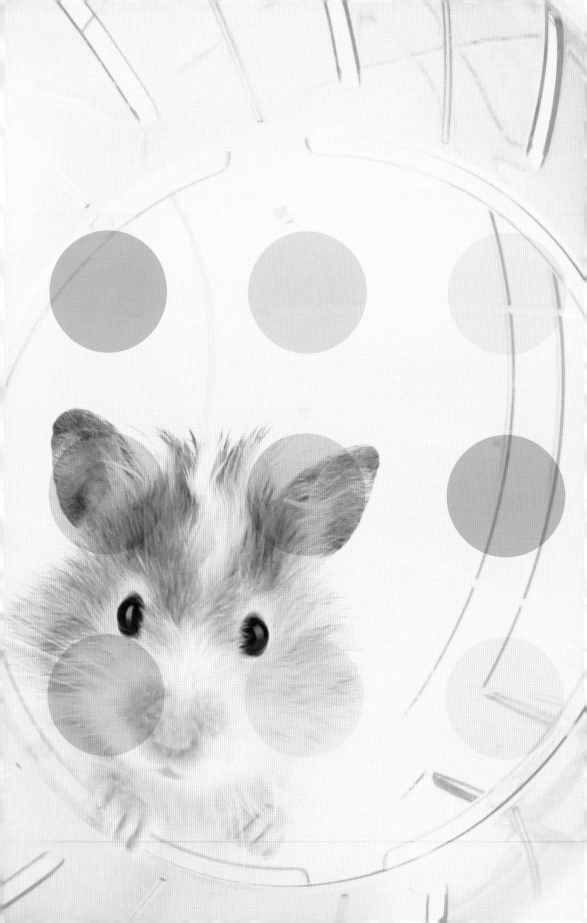

04
WEIGHT MANAGEMENT CLINICS

PREVENTION AND CONTROL METHODS WITH A SPECIFIC LINK BETWEEN OWNER AND PRACTITIONER

When weight management programmes are considered, the first ones that come to mind are the human-based, very well advertised ones, such as Slimming World and Weight Watchers®. The biggest consideration for a person who is managing weight clinics and programmes is the acknowledgement from owners. If an owner does not identify that their animal is overweight, then this is the big issue.

To be able to effectively manage a weight programme, we have to consider a variety of factors to ensure the effectiveness of the programme.

WEIGHT MANAGEMENT CLINICS

Weight management clinics can be very effective when run from a veterinary practice or pet store. Helping owners and patients can be very rewarding for animal and veterinary nursing staff, leading to job satisfaction.

Staff that take part and manage weight clinics should be passionate about the subject. If it is evident that the passion about weight management is missing, then the client will not follow the designated set programme. Veterinary professionals or animal practitioners must be competent and have the skillset needed to manage a weight programme; it is also important for the company to invest in and support this type of service.

Communication is one of the most important employee attributes when managing programmes which require active participation from members of the public. Effective communication is one of the most critical components of customer service for an organisation. Customer service efforts are designed to ensure that all customers have prompt and efficient delivery of their individualized needs. Also, the practitioner will need to be adequately prepared to deal with complaints, so training and support must be provided.

Staff involved in managing the weight clinic must be aware of their non-verbal communication and how this comes across to clients. Staff must be assertive and attentive to clients and display open body language so that they are able to effectively show that they are listening. It is important to make the client feel valued, which will increase the likelihood of commitment to the programme.

Effective communication to clients requires a thorough understanding of the client's needs and perspective outcomes. Sometimes, it also may be beneficial to get consumer feedback, possibly via a survey.

Staff must accept that there will be limitations to their role and they must know when to refer a client on when they are unable to deal with the client's needs themselves. Commitment to a customer service standard is important for customer satisfaction and loyalty.

SETTING UP AND PREPARING FOR WEIGHT MANAGEMENT PROGRAMMES

The first part of the journey is to choose the most appropriate name for the weight management programme. The name must be appealing to draw in new clients and memorable for existing clients to promote the business by word of mouth. Human names must be avoided due to copyright potentials. Some of the brands of pet food have materials that can be extremely valuable if used correctly. Sometimes the organisation will need to develop their own resources for a more personalized and bespoke service, which is also a good marketing tool.

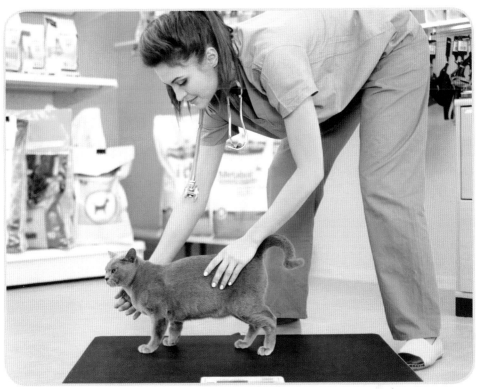

↱ Pet weight clinic.
Photo: Adobe Stock – Nejron Photo

ADVERTISING YOUR PROGRAMME

Finding the right clientele for the clinics

Once the clinics have been planned and established then appropriate advertising can be adopted to promote the service to its target audience. Identifying typical clients is another activity that needs to be completed before advertising to maximize recruitment. Once the advertisement has been placed, you should keep a register of clients' details who would like to participate in the programme. In the instance where the company has a known client base it can be beneficial to send out an email or sms invitation to the programme or an appointment reminder. Staff need to be discreet and considerate

HANDY HINT
CLIENTS' DETAILS

Name, telephone number, email, animal details, location, availability for clinics, date of enquiry and follow-up date, staff details

○ ○ ○

47

when counselling clients on the referral of their pet to the weight management programme as some clients may take time to accept and come around to the idea.

Ensure the paraphernalia has the specific details and times for the programmes and that this information is shared with clients appropriately and with plenty of notice so they can make arrangements for attendance and finance. Advanced notice also gives plenty of time for clients to make enquiries and ask questions prior to the event. Everyone now has access to the internet, therefore information should be published online with a well-managed frequently asked questions section. The company should make clear their protocol for response to enquiries to ensure client expectations are met.

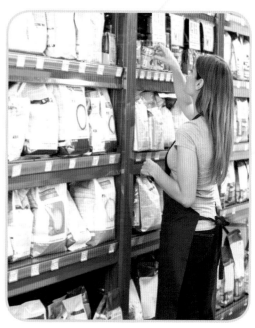

↘ Pet food packets at store.
Photo: Adobe Stock – Tyler Olson

PLANNING AND MANAGEMENT OF THE WEIGHT MANAGEMENT CLINICS

Each clinic or programme will require a specific plan; this is to ensure standardization between clients and staff.

Weight clinic appointment

The allocated time for the initial appointment should be reflective of the extensive discussion with the owner to ensure a detailed history and full understanding of the animal's daily routine; follow-up appointments may not take as long. It is important that as much information as possible is gained to fully understand the reasons why the animal is overweight.

Ensure that the scales are calibrated before getting the animal on the scales. It is advisable to weigh the animal at the same time if possible for the programme to avoid excuses, such as, 'he has just eaten his breakfast'.

Use a tape measure. It can be advisable to give one to each owner so they can see the difference themselves.

Take measurements from the animal's neck, chest and abdomen. This is really helpful to encourage owners and get them to take responsibility for the programme. It is also something tangible, where they can see the difference.

Ensure that the measurements are completed at the same area each time, to ensure validity of the results. It is useful to have digital images to show the differences and changes in weight.

Ensure that the information gained covers the quantity, timing and type of food that the animal is being fed. Also, enquire whether the animal has any special treats throughout the day.

Careful questioning may be needed to remind owners that even a little biscuit before bedtime is classified as a treat. Comprehensive understanding of the animal's exercise regime must be gained: whether a dog is walked on the lead, off the lead, the duration and frequency.

Questions to be asked

- The animal's daily routine: how many times a day it is fed? What is its level and intensity of exercise?
- How long is the animal left for, does it go to pet care, does someone pop in and see it when left alone?
- Does anyone else in the house feed the pet? Are there children in the house who might drop food or feed the pet?
- If it is an outdoor cat, do the owners have knowledge of it going next door for food? Or is it a hunter?

When this information has been gained you will have a clearer idea why the animal is overweight and how to carefully advise and agree with the owner a new management regime. To increase compliance, it is imperative that the owner shows acknowledgment that their animal is overweight before you commence a weight management programme.

Then commence a body condition score (BCS). Owners like to be able to see the information in front of them. Give them the details of how you complete the BCS and get them to complete on their own as well (see page 8).

Courcier (2010) identified that owners find it challenging to accurately BCS a cat, especially if they are long-haired.

At this point, the method of delivery will be different for every owner. The owner's characteristics will need to be considered. The owners must be made aware of the significant risks of obesity and its effects on animal health and physiological state. But they must also be made aware of their need to improve the animal's exercise and lifestyle. An effective weight reduction programme requires full commitment from both staff members and owners. Animal records need to be clear and consistent and contain all the information discussed at the patient's visits. They must contain the key details of the management programme, for example amount/type of food, exercise, appointments, targets and measurements. There should also be a goal set for the intended timeframe.

Competitions

There is nothing more motivating than a little healthy competition. Create a slimmer of the month certificate and give rewards. Many brands will have big competitions and it may be beneficial to enter the owner and animal in an appropriate one. An incentive would be a free gift (toy, diet food, etc.) to the animal that wins slimmer of the month and a big gift for slimmer of the year. Ensure these are visible within the workplace as they will encourage other owners to partake in the challenge.

FEEDING A REDUCING DIET

Reducing diets are the most effective method to be used in combination with a weight management programme. It may require a veterinary professional to decide the most suitable diet for the weight management programme. The key is to reduce weight, but this must be in a controlled health manner. There are many reducing diets within the pet food market which are designed to aid weight loss by providing the required nutrients but reducing the calories and making the animal feel satiated (full). Reducing the animal's current diet will not ensure that the animal is receiving its required nutritional demands as reducing food will reduce volume of intake of nutrients. So, a weight-reducing diet would be seen to be more beneficial and better from a nutritional point of view for the animal. Specific medical conditions or allergies must also be considered when providing diet choices. This will require discussion with the consulting veterinary surgeon. If the diet is to be changed, manufacturer's recommendations for diet change must be followed to prevent gastrointestinal upset.

ANIMAL EXERCISE

An appropriate diet on its own will not contribute to a good weight management programme; it requires a combination of measures. The age of the animal, breed and the type of exercise it is given needs careful consideration. Pre-existing medical or orthopaedic problems may affect the amount or type of exercise that can be given. The time of year may affect the animal's programme as during the summer months consideration will need to be given to the possibility of heat stroke when exercising. Also, some owners will not exercise animals when weather conditions are poor, so consideration must be given to exercise and play that can be given inside.

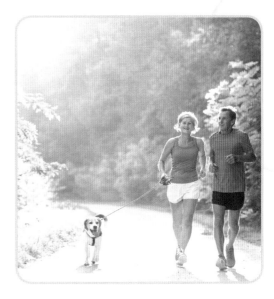

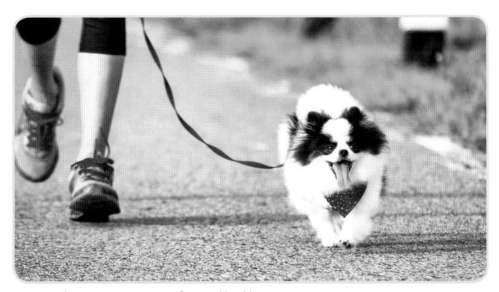

↘ Daily exercise is important for good health.
Photo: Adobe Stock – Halfpoint; analysis121980

Additional forms of exercise can be suitable for some dogs depending on age, breed and health status:

○ A gentle game of fetch with a ball, frisbee or tug rope can be fun and rewarding
○ Take the dog running: start off power walking and gradually increase the speed and duration over time
○ Flyball can be really useful for intelligent and high-energy breeds; there are clubs that can be used
○ Agility can be a good way to provide mental stimulation and is fun for both the dog and owner; children can also be involved
○ Hydrotherapy is a really effective way of using exercise with minimal body force; this could be useful for geriatric or arthritic animals that are happy to be in water
○ Puzzle toys and games are challenging and make the animal work harder for its food
○ A gentle game of chase can be fun for any animal and will help to increase heart rate
○ Off-lead running can be really good as long as the animal is adequately trained and the recall is good
○ Join a fitness class for owner and dog – there are various classes in local areas. Dog yoga is now a thing!

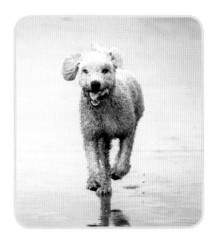

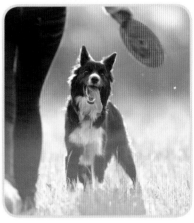

↘ Make exercise fun with a gentle game of ball or Frisbee.
Photo: Adobe Stock – dazb75; adamfichna

↘ Puzzle toys can create stimulating entertainment.
Photo: Adobe Stock – alexei_tm

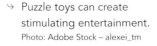

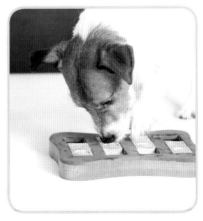

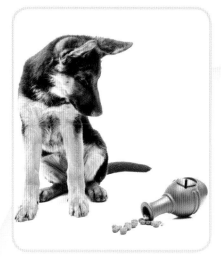

↳ Creating a challenge can be
  rewarding and encourages the
  animal to be active.
  Photo: Adobe Stock – Roman Milert

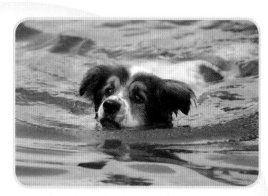

↳ Regular swimming in safe water
  is a fun form of exercise.
  Photo: Adobe Stock – dejavudesigns

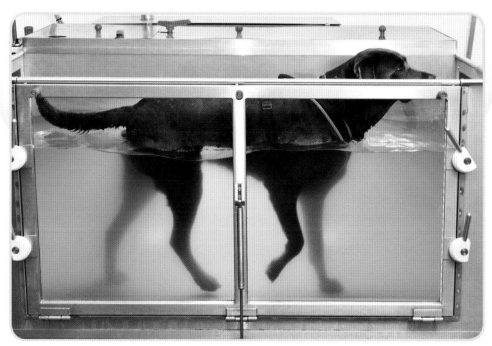

↳ Hydrotherapy is a non-weight-bearing therapy that can be used to
  promote preoperative or general fitness, aid postoperative recovery
  and provide relief from chronic conditions.
  Photo: Adobe Stock – Christoph Hähnel

Here are some suggestions for additional exercise for cats:

○ Get a laser light and encourage the cat to chase this in the house
○ Use a secure harness and lead and walk outside
○ Hide food around the house so that they have to actively seek the food; cats are a natural foraging species so this can encourage natural behaviours
○ Use stick toys to encourage play and jumping
○ Battery-powered furry mice to chase around the house
○ Use various size boxes to encourage hiding and jumping
○ Cat climbing trees and post climbers
○ Cat puzzle toys.

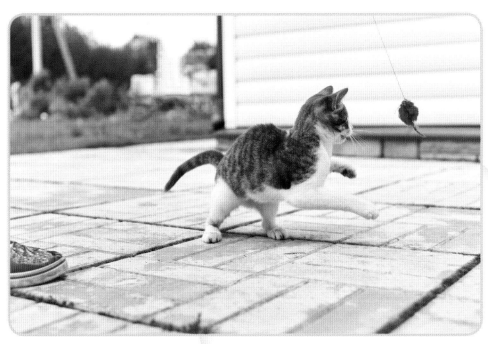

↳ Think of creative ways to encourage activity and promote natural behaviours.
Photo: Adobe Stock – Artem

Here are some suggestions for additional exercise for rabbits:

○ Daily opportunities to run outside the hutch in a safe part of the garden or house
○ Toys, for example plastic toys: they like to pick these up and play with them
○ Paper: roll into a ball for the rabbit to chase in a similar way to fetch play
○ Logic toys
○ Gnawing block
○ Tunnels
○ Allowing an area for the rabbit to dig, ensuring it is safe and will not escape
○ Daily handling and socialization with owner.

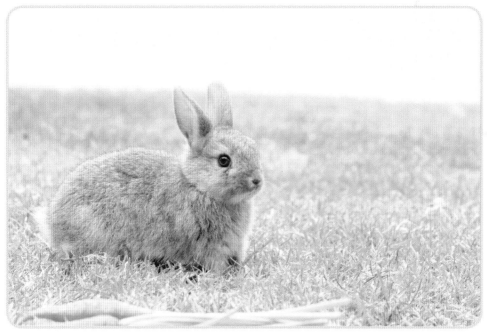

↱ Daily exercise and time out of the hutch is important for the pet rabbit.
Photo: Adobe Stock – takorn

↘ A hamster may enjoy a
ten-minute play in a ball.
Photo: Adobe Stock - Africa
Studio

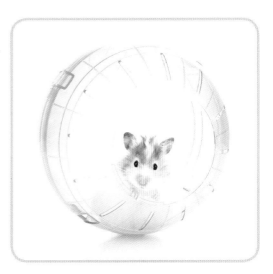

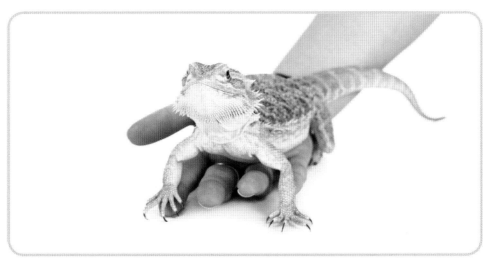

↘ Time out of the vivarium is important for reptiles.
Photo: Adobe Stock – adogslifephoto

APPROPRIATE DIETS

One of the most important things for the animal is the diet change. Owners need
to understand that the diet is not removing the method of treating. A good piece
of advice would be to reduce the proportion of the daily allocated diet and allocate
this for treating. You could also look at behavioural modification, removing the
treating system altogether and rewarding with play and toys. A good treat for a cat
is a toy or some catnip. When using the appropriate diet that has been chosen for
the weight-reducing programme, it is a good idea to weigh and measure the food

and to show the owner, so they know how much to feed. It can be beneficial to weigh the daily amount of food in the morning and keep the food in a container; any rewards given during the day can come out of the container which will prevent offering additional food items and thus overfeeding.

The optical illusion theory (Delboeuf) and the size–contrast illusion (Ebbinghaus-Titchener) describe an owner's perception that he or she is feeding his or her dog more, just by using a smaller bowl.

When the consultation has finished, it is imperative that the owner understands the key aims and benefits of the programme created. Ensure they have had the opportunity to ask appropriate questions, no matter how small or silly the question might seem. Ensure that the owner has been encouraged to be committed and agree on a course of action, the day and time to attend. Book the next appointment and ensure that the owner has all the appropriate paperwork and BCS information. Ensure that the digital image of the animal and the relevant measurements have been taken.

When following up on the programme, ensure that the animal is aiming to lose 1–2% of body weight per week (maximum 1.3% for cats; Harvey and Taylor, 2012). The targeted weight loss will be given on an individual basis and this can be tracked on the paperwork that is provided. If no weight loss has occurred, effective questioning will need to be used to find the reasoning behind this. The weight management programme may require amendments to ensure that some weight loss can be achieved. Plot the information on a graph so that even a small amount will be evident and visible for the owners to recognise.

Hopefully, this chapter has given enough information to personalize a weight management clinic. This can be amended to fit individual clients and pets. It is extremely important to ensure the continued commitment of the owners is evident. It is also important that staff members completing the clinic are enthusiastic and driven about the management of obesity.

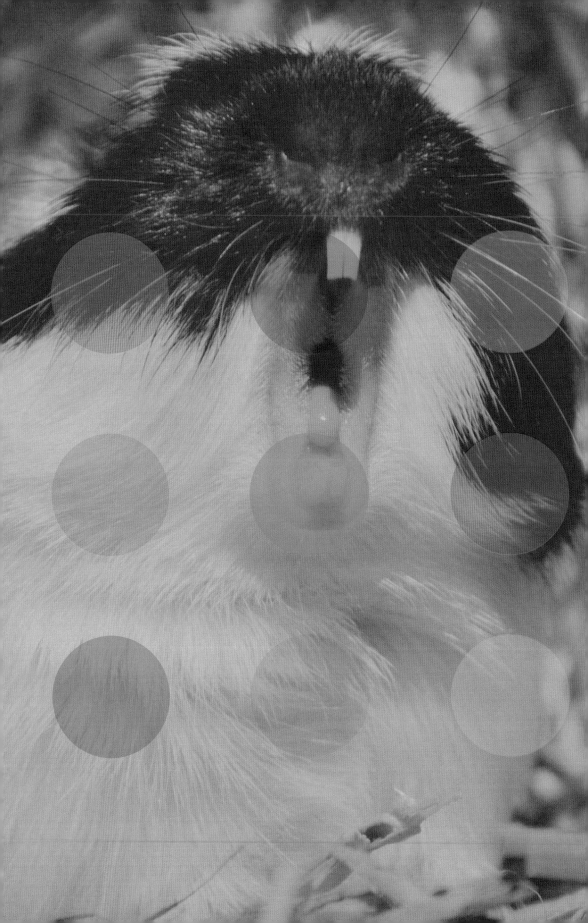

05

DIET-RELATED DISEASE

○ ○ ○

AN ANIMAL'S HEALTH will reflect the quality of diet given. Responsible pet guardians should carefully research dietary requirements specific to the species, life stage and health. Senior animals are more predisposed to diet-related disease due to the ageing of their digestive system and organs which does not allow for effective absorption of nutrients. There are a number of diseases that can occur due to incorrect nutrition. This is why it is extremely important for pet guardians to understand what is going in an animal's food and what requirements they may have at different life stages. Educating pet carers is the way to providing better nutrition to animals.

There are many diseases that can be a result of incorrect nutrition and feeding plans. This chapter will discuss just a few of them.

DIETARY DEFICIENCY AND TOXICITY

○ Are generally rare and usually associated with neglect or by feeding an unbalanced diet.
○ Disease states, usually of the intestinal system, can lead to deficiencies in some or all dietary components.

Diseases that cause malnutrition and weight loss can be grouped into one of four headings:

○ Lack of nutrient intake (inappetence or dysphagia)
○ Lack of nutrient absorption (vomiting, diarrhoea, small intestinal disease, exocrine pancreatic insufficiency)
○ Cachectic state (increased nutrient demand in animals with a variety of disease, e.g. neoplasia, congestive heart failure, hyperthyroidism)
○ Excessive nutrient loss, e.g. protein-losing nephropathy, diabetes mellitus, protein-losing enteropathy.

OBESITY

Obesity is now one of the more common diseases seen in veterinary practice. Obesity itself is a horrid, controllable disease. It should also be noted that obesity causes many of the other diseases discussed in this chapter.

The biggest issue with pet obesity is getting the owner to recognize that their animal is obese. Many owners fail to recognize this, thinking the animal is within the normal recommended weight for the breed. Owner compliance is key in dealing with this disease.

Owners need to be educated about the caloric values within food and the impact of little treats or titbits.

Although reducing calories will aid in dealing with obesity, the owner also needs to increase exercise for their animal. Diet will not on its own reduce the animal's weight.

Obesity can cause:

○ Heart disease
○ Urinary disorders
○ Arthritis
○ Diabetes
○ Cancers.

This is just a small list of key disorders which are caused by or have increased risk factors for obesity. There are many others which can be caused by or have higher risk factors from obesity.

See Chapter 4 for the management of obesity.

HEART DISEASE

There are numerous causes of heart disease and they can often be breed-specific. Unfortunately, due to various factors there are predisposing genetics in relation to heart conditions. One of the key factors that requires consideration is the sodium (salt) content in an animal's diet.

High levels of salt in diets of mainly dogs and cats can cause excess water retention in blood vessels resulting in elevated blood pressure. This continued elevated blood pressure causes increased pressure on the heart and the heart enlarges to overcome this increased pressure. This can cause various heart disorders that will require veterinary attention. Table scraps fed to animals may be high in salt and should not be recommended as a nice little treat. There are various diets available for animals with heart disease or predisposed disorders. There are also diets which have a monitored level of sodium.

URINARY DISORDERS

Diets can have numerous impacts on urinary disorders. The different pH balance of foods may cause urinary calculi and crystals. Obese middle-aged male cats have a prevalence of urinary crystals, mainly struvite. This can be managed and controlled by changes in the diet and lifestyle of the animal. Different urinary calculi are caused by overexposure to minerals within the diet, calcium oxalate crystals being mainly composed of calcium and another common urinary crystal, struvite, being primarily composed of magnesium and phosphorus.

Urinary disorders can be extremely dangerous if left untreated. If you suspect that your animal may be suffering from any form of urinary discomfort you should seek veterinary attention.

When an animal is diagnosed with a urinary disorder, there are different diets available to reduce the recurrence of calculi or crystals. These are usually prescribed by veterinary surgeons. Diet changes should be completed by introducing the new diet in small amounts, gradually reducing the old diet, to reduce gastric upset. This must be completed with someone who has knowledge, as giving an animal the incorrect pH balance of food could exacerbate existing issues! The animal's water intake should also be monitored and it may be that the veterinary surgeon will change the animal onto a moist diet to increase water consumption.

DIARRHOEA

Diet change is one of the most common causes of pet diarrhoea. Owners should be advised when they are changing a diet that the process should be completed slowly and over a long period of time, gradually increasing the new diet and decreasing the old diet. When an animal has acute or chronic diarrhoea other factors will need consideration. Chronic diarrhoea has many causes, one of which is small intestine microbial overgrowth. Acute diarrhoea is usually a result of infections, parasites or toxins. Stress can be a precursor to diarrhoea, especially in small domestic animals such as hamsters. Food intolerances and allergies will also need careful consideration especially if the diarrhoea continues for an extended period.

There are many protocols that can be put in place when an animal has diarrhoea but it is advisable to seek veterinary attention at all times.

FOOD ALLERGIES

These are also discussed within other chapters in this book.

Food allergies can account for a significant number of patients seen in a veterinary practice with allergy signs. Some of the key signs of food allergies include diarrhoea, vomiting, pruritus, erythema and swollen ears and paws. There are many different types of food allergies, some of the most common being beef and chicken: these are foods that are regularly used as flavouring in most pet foods. Also, the quality of the food may cause some allergic reactions, especially if the food is filled with grains, cereals and bulking agents.

It is important if an animal could be considered to have a food allergy, that veterinary attention is sought and the animal most likely placed on a dietary management programme.

CASE STUDY

JASPER

Jasper is a male neutered springer spaniel who lives a very active life with his pet parent. He was fed on a chicken-based, formulated, complete dry kibble diet. His pet parent noted repeated ear infections and noticed he was chewing his feet and tail. Following a discussion with his owner and a veterinary professional it was decided to introduce a grain free diet. The new diet was gradually introduced over a 14 day period and 12 months on the occurrence of ear infections, feet and tail chewing has been practically eliminated. It was noticed within a few months that his occurrences of ear-based infections had dramatically decreased and his chewing of his feet and tail had reduced.

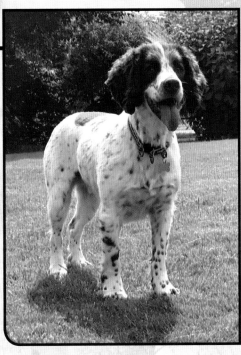

↳ Jasper.
Photo: Helen Coleman

DENTAL ISSUES

One of the biggest issues that many pet guardians have with their animals is their bad breath! This is termed halitosis. There are many different causes for dental disease, some of which some can be prevented. Tooth decay causes halitosis and can also cause discomfort to your pet. A type of bacteria that lives on teeth gets its energy from starches in the animal's diet. These bacteria form together and are known as plaque. They produce an acid which rots the tooth, causing tooth abscesses and resulting bad breath. If this dental change is left untreated then there will be resulting tooth decay and possibly tooth loss. Animals should be provided with methods and health care to promote healthy teeth and gums. Pet guardians should provide the animal with dental chews and ways to maintain oral hygiene. Care should be taken to select healthy dental chews that are not full of sugar and additives. For dogs and cats there should be a daily effort to clean the teeth and gums with a species-specific toothpaste and brush. This of course can be difficult for owners to achieve so a dental procedure at the vets is probable if preventative methods are not practiced from an early age. It should be noted that a high-quality diet and avoidance of feeding table scraps can also promote good dental health. The provision of bones is a natural plaque prevention method; and although there is currently little evidence to support their effectiveness, powder supplements can be added to food which claim to prevent the build-up of plaque and if not treated will harden to form tartar. Unfortunately,

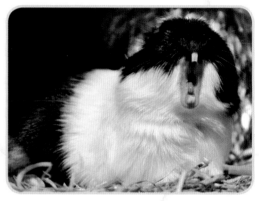

↳ Open routed teeth.
Photo: Pixabay

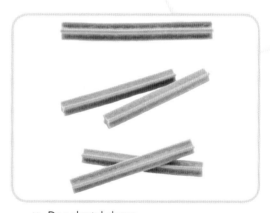

↳ Dog dental chews.
Photo: Adobe Stock – amstockphoto

some dog breeds such as brachycephalic (short-nosed) dogs are predisposed to tartar build-up due to poor alignment of teeth and miniature breeds can experience teeth misalignment. Rabbits and some small rodents have open routed teeth which means their teeth continue to grow; the teeth are kept to a normal length by ingestion of species-specific diets and the provision of gnawing blocks. There are diets specific for dogs and cats that have been formulated to aid in the prevention of dental disease.

DIETARY NUTRITION-RELATED DEFICIENCIES

Some pet guardians have the idea that their animal should be fed a diet that is high in muscle meat and organ tissue: this should not be the case. A high meat and organ diet can cause a disease termed nutritional-related secondary hyperparathyroidism, which is caused by the diet fed being high in phosphorus but low in calcium. The body reacts to a reduction in bone mineralization, and to maintain homeostasis, releases hormone responses that return the calcium phosphorus ratio within normal ranges. This increases the absorption of calcium from the intestines and reabsorption within the bones. This results in the bones being inadequately mineralized and can cause skeletal diseases such as rickets and osteomalacia.

Rickets occurs in growing animals that have inadequate calcium in their diet; the long bones of the animal will bow and end up with enlarged ends. This can result in permanent deformity in the animal.

Osteomalacia occurs in older animals who have a lack of calcium in their diet, resulting in the bones becoming softer and some pathological fractures may be seen.

Certain binding agents such as oxalate that may be added to foods, can also affect the absorption of calcium from the diet.

Vitamin D is actively involved in the absorption of calcium; this is usually provided at the required amount in nutritionally-balanced diets, however, the levels may be lower in home-made or poor-quality diets with lots of cereals. If these diets are fed, there will be evident low blood calcium levels known as hypocalcaemia.

Protein deficiency

When offering a diet to a carnivorous or omnivorous animal, it is important to recognize the protein source and quality. Although rarely seen, a lack of protein can result in the following:

○ Poor growth, skin lesions
○ Weight loss, poor appetite
○ Impaired immune function, healing and repair
○ Loss of coat condition (rough and dull)
○ Hypoproteinaemia.

Protein excess

○ Can be used for energy or stored as adipose tissue.
○ Ammonia removed from protein is converted to urea by the liver and excreted via the kidneys.
○ Excess amounts of urea can overwork the kidneys and can cause damage.

Vitamin A deficiency

This can result from a diet reduced in fat or in animals that have digestive diseases resulting in disorders in absorption of fat:

○ Can result in poor skin and coat condition
○ Dry or greasy coat
○ Flaky skin
○ Build-up of scurf in the coat.

Essential fatty acids

These play a very important role in the animal's diet: if animals are suffering from liver or fat absorption disorders then they may require supplementation. Essential fatty acids are responsible for maintaining healthy coat and skin, immunity and wound healing.

Magnesium deficiency

This may occur during times of extreme stress or if the animal is suffering from a disease which is causing an increased urine output.

○ This can cause muscle weakness and can result in a lack of thiamin (part of the vitamin B group) which can then cause disorders of the central nervous system.

Cats are known as obligate carnivores which means that they absolutely must have meat provided in their diet. If a cat is fed a diet deficient in animal protein, it can suffer from the following deficiencies:

○ Taurine (often seen in cats fed dog or vegetarian diets)
○ Feline central retinal degeneration, impaired immune function, poor reproduction, abnormalities in kittens, dilated cardiomyopathy
○ Arachidonic acid
○ Niacin.

Cats also require selenium/vitamin E. A diet deficient in this can result in a disease termed steatitis or yellow fat disease. This is the fat cells dying and can be extremely painful in the cat.

CASE STUDY

BERNARD

Bernard is a 9-year-old male neutered Cavalier King Charles spaniel. His pet guardian had noticed that he had become off colour and food obsessed to the extent he had started to invade the bin and its contents. This was a dramatic change in his feeding behaviour. He was also suffering with a case of borborygmic, excessive intestinal sounds. On presentation to the veterinary clinic, the veterinary surgeon could not see anything significant on his health check. It was advised he had a full blood test taken. This included a full haematology and biochemistry profile and main vitamin tests. When the results were received it was noticed that his vitamin B levels were very low. He immediately started injectable vitamin B. It should be noted that this was thought to be from a small microbial overgrowth in his small intestine caused by a bad case of diarrhoea. He was put on medication to control the growth and for control of the good intestinal bacteria. He was significantly improved within a few months of starting his treatment.

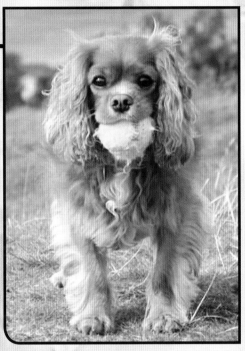

↪ Bernard.
Photo: Tony Keegan

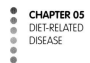
ARTHRITIS

Arthritis is defined as inflammation of the joint surface. This is commonly seen in older animals. Unfortunately, due to the high prevalence of obesity in domesticated species, arthritis is not just a disease of elderly animals. If an animal is diagnosed with this disease, obesity management may need to be considered if it is overweight. There are various dietary supplements available such as glucosamine and green-lipped mussel extract. These aid in reducing inflammation and pain from arthritis and degenerative joint disease.

PANCREATITIS

This is a disease which in itself is extremely painful. The pancreas becomes inflamed and leaks digestive enzymes which cause the pancreas to self-digest. It can be both chronic and acute. Both forms can be life-threatening and can make the animal extremely unwell. A common cause of pancreatitis is a sudden change of diet or exposure to a very fatty food. It can be seen at Christmas time in emergency vets when the animals are fed treats high in fat. Unfortunately, it can also be classified as an idiopathic disease which means that it can be of no apparent cause.

TABLE 5.1
DIFFERENTIATION BETWEEN ACUTE AND CHRONIC PANCREATITIS

PANCREATIC DISEASE	POSSIBLE CAUSES	CLINICAL SIGNS
Acute	Obesity	High temperature
	Trauma	Vomiting
	Surgical operations	Abdominal pain
	High-fat diets	Dehydration
		Collapse
		Shock
Chronic	Idiopathic	Anorexia
	Infections	Vague pain signs
		Depression
		Weight loss

Animals suffering from this and in recovery will require significant dietary changes. The animal should start off on a high carbohydrate diet which has the least stimulating effect on the pancreatic enzymes. When returned to eating normally, the animal should be fed a diet which is easy digestible, low-fat and reduced in protein by a high biological value. This will require support, tests and intense veterinary care and services.

DIABETES

Diabetes is a prevalent disease in the veterinary practice. There is a genetic consideration with diabetes but there is significant evidence that obesity has a role in the increase of this disease.

Diabetes itself stops the animal from regulating its own blood sugar levels. Usually this has an immune link in dogs and an obesity link in both dogs and cats. It is seen more commonly in middle-aged, obese, male cats.

Diabetic animals will need significant dietary management which will be given alongside medicinal/veterinary support and treatments. It is very important to remember that if an animal is on a diabetic protocol, the diet should not be changed too quickly and consideration will need to be given as to when the animal has had its last food. This is a disease which will require commitment from owners as the management has key protocols. High-sugar treats and readily available sugars such as cereals should be avoided and the animal will most likely be recommended to go onto a prescription diet to complement therapy.

BLOAT AND TORSION

These illnesses can strike very suddenly in dogs of any age, although deep-chested and large, active breeds suffer most commonly. Symptoms can include extreme restlessness, salivation, successful or unsuccessful vomiting and progressive abdominal swelling. Unless spotted very quickly, these symptoms can lead to severe shock and death in as few as six hours from the onset. Irreparable damage can be caused to the dog's internal organs even if the symptoms are spotted quickly, due to shock, which can severely complicate treatment. Should your dog show any of the above signs it is imperative that you seek veterinary assistance as soon as possible. In the case of torsion, the immediate decompression of the stomach is vital, and surgery will be required if the dog is suffering from bloat.

Torsion occurs when the stomach becomes swollen as a result of bloat, and then rotates causing a loss of circulation to the stomach and other organs.

Most of the research into the causes of bloat have been inconclusive. There are a few suspected causes (such as exercising after meals or consuming a large amount of water after eating a large meal of dried food) but there are still a number of likely causes which have not been discounted. These include sudden changes in diet, vaccinations or exposure to high-stress situations.

EXOCRINE PANCREATIC INSUFFICIENCY

A condition caused by insufficient production or total loss of pancreatic enzymes resulting in the inability to adequately digest fat and, to a lesser extent, protein and carbohydrates in the diet, resulting in maldigestion. It is commonly a congenital problem, usually because the pancreas fails to develop normally. It is also a disease that animals can get over time; in dogs, this is usually due to damage of the pancreas; it is rare in cats.

Clinical signs include:

○ Polyphagia
○ Coprophagia
○ Weight loss
○ Diarrhoea
○ Steatorrhoea (excess fat in faeces)
○ Flatulence
○ Poor hair coat.

This animal will require very specific nutritional management and is best transitioned onto a diet that is digestible, low-fat, high biological value protein and with reduced fibre. The animal will need to be continually monitored by a veterinary surgeon as it will require medical treatment

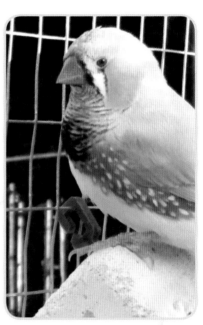

↳ Zebra finch sitting on an iodine block.
Photo: Darren Gibson

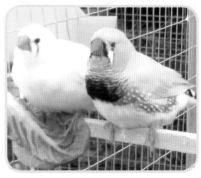

↳ Zebra finches and fresh food.
Photo: Darren Gibson

and supportive supplements to ensure the animal is absorbing the nutrients correctly.

COMMON PROBLEMS OF BIRDS

These are discussed in greater detail in Chapter 11. Bird nutrition is very specific and bird owners must be given enough information so that they can make an educated choice on feeding their birds. Below are some of the most common nutritional diseases of birds:

- ○ Hypovitaminosis A: causes upper respiratory disease, swelling of eyes and nasal discharge
- ○ Hypovitaminosis B: causes poor feather quality and lesions of the mouth and skin
- ○ Calcium deficiency: causes drooping wings, inactivity and soft shells
- ○ Iodine deficiency: causes breathing difficulties, enlarged thyroid gland and loss of voice
- ○ Hypovitaminosis C: causes increased susceptibility to infections, slow wound healing and general debilitation.

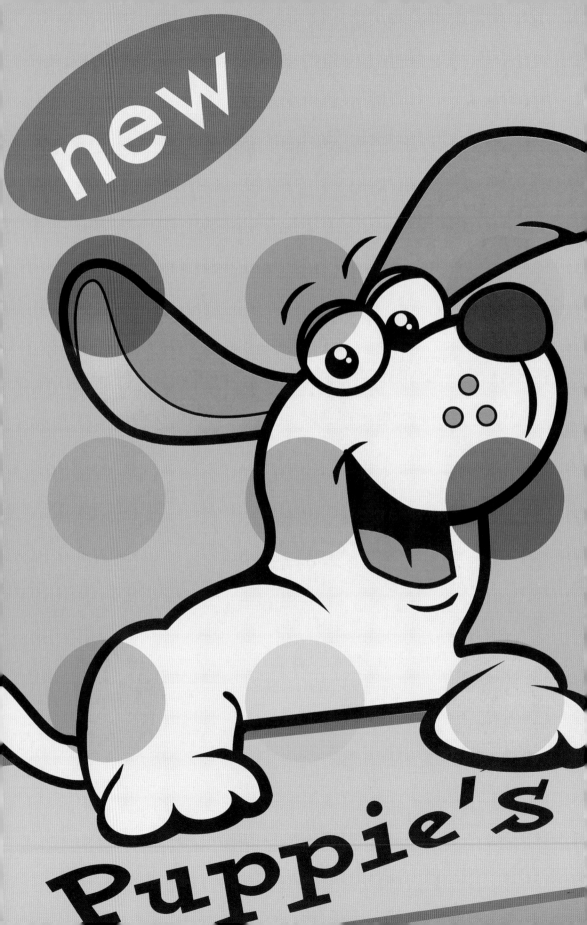

06
MARKETING AND
CONSUMER BEHAVIOUR

THERE ARE specific regulations governing the sale of animal food.

These are:

○ The Animal Feed (Composition, Marketing and Use) (England) Regulations 2015
○ The Animal Feed (Hygiene, Sampling etc. and Enforcement) (England) Regulations 2015.

The regulations stipulate the level of information that should be included on pet food labels in relation to content of the food and additives. It also allows for the enforcement of other types of EU-led legislation (PFMA, 2015).

The Pet Food Manufacturers Association is the leading trade body for the UK pet industry. Their aim is to provide a balanced regulatory environment for the production of nutritious and safe food. Also, they are key advocates for responsible pet ownership. They provide key information to members of the public and also have a lead role in forming opinions regarding pet food manufacture throughout the EU. Additionally, in the US the Pet Food Institute (PFI) promotes innovation for the safe production or nutritious pet food; further ensuring pet owners are educated in health and nutrition.

The European Pet Food Industry Federation, FEDIAF represent the pet food industry from many European countries and institutions. They are part of a committee that is striving for legislation guidelines for pet food and aim to construct a legislation framework for the production of safe, nutritious and palatable pet food (FEDIAF, 2015).

The Pet Industry Federation (PIF) is a membership association for pet industry specialists. It is a hallmark of quality to be a PIF member as all members agree to follow sector-specific charters to demonstrate good practice (PIF, 2015). The above associations focus on the trademark and quality of pet food that is manufactured and supplied within the EU.

We will now look at the advertising of pet food. The primary modes of advertising are television, supermarkets, veterinary practices and industry-relevant magazines and leaflets.

Choices made by pet owners are not necessarily based on nutritional value, but what looks good and often more considered from a humanistic view. Television usually has the most profound impact as the visual advertisement focusses on the ability to influence the owner's choice. The food is presented to resonate with humans, appeal to our anthropomorphic tendencies and influence our brand preference. It uses a series of bright, colourful adverts which portray the animal in a happy environment, enjoying its food.

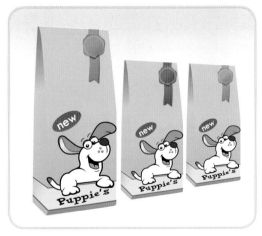

Advertising within retail outlets must make an immediate impact; there is less time to 'tell the story' therefore imagery must capture the 'moment' to draw attention to the brand. This type of advertising can often

↘ Advertising.
Photo: Adobe Stock – Maximo Sanz

be overwhelming and confusing for the consumer who will not necessarily make the most informed choice when selecting the brand of food. Pet owners do not necessarily know what to look for when choosing the right brand of food which is how they can be drawn in by advertising. Clever placement of products along with expert branding make convenient shopping for impulse buyers, who may not necessarily question the quality of food, over the packaging, branding and price. Many owners are influenced by the packaging, for example if there is an image of a specific breed of dog, owners with the same breed of dog may be drawn to the product regardless of the product content.

It is relatively typical over recent years to find a range of brands from value to premium within supermarkets that strive to provide choice for the consumer. Consumer choice is important, which is why many pet food manufacturers offer varying levels of product quality and value to suit different socioeconomic states. This in turn at least encourages consumers to link brand, price and value.

Brands and the cost of pet food go hand in hand. Manufacturers often have to compromise on the quality of ingredients to keep costs down, hence a greater range of cost-effective foods are available to customers. Technically, this is a false economy as it is commonplace to use grains to bulk out the food and these will be of low quality, therefore the caregiver will have to feed a larger proportion per feed in order to provide necessary levels of energy. A higher-energy, dense food is likely to be more expensive since the type of carbohydrates is often rice or potato rather than cheap cereals. Furthermore, the protein source is less likely to be derivative-based with higher-grade meat used instead which obviously comes with higher production costs which are naturally passed on to the consumer. Grain free diets is a more recent phenomenon which contain less carbohydrate and more protein which are considered more nutritionally valuable and easily digested. Premium foods are not something to be wary of – you get what you pay for – but second, the amount of food fed per portion is often less to account for the higher-

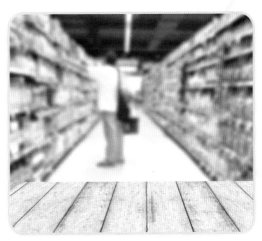

↘ Price branding and marketing.
Photo: Adobe Stock – Kwangmoo

quality ingredients which makes the overall purchase more cost-effective than it first appears. Although, there are certain brands that label themselves as premium food when actually it is more a case of clever marketing and packaging. This is another reason why it is important to understand the nutritional analysis, so that the consumer is able to make informed decisions based on quality as opposed to the initial price.

Low-cost foods will have additional ingredients to increase palatability to compensate for low-grade ingredients. Hence, the salt and fat content is often higher in these types of food which long term can be detrimental to health. The question to ask is whether the initial cost of food is worth compromising the health of the animal with the increased likelihood of vet bills later in life.

FASHION FEEDING

Social media can have a huge impact on diet choice for owners. Many celebrities will link themselves and advocate different diet types such as vegan, grain-free, hypoallergenic and natural. Education to owners must be there to guide their choice and ensure the influence is appropriate and will continue to provide their animal with a nutritionally-balanced diet according to its life stage and species.

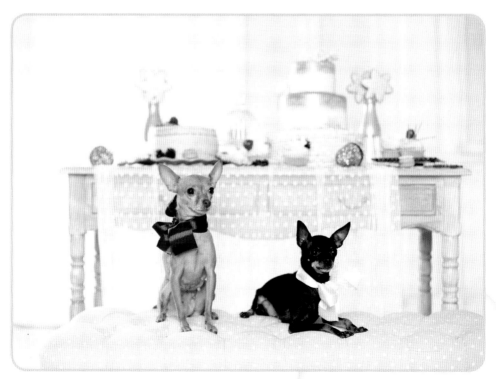

↳ Fashion feeding.
Photo: Adobe Stock – olga guzhevnikova

FLAVOUR ENHANCERS AND COLOURS/SHAPES

These are specifically put into diets and are cleverly advertised to influence the anthropomorphic mindset in animal owners: 'That food has gravy in it, I love gravy on my dinner'. Again, with careful support, advice and education owners can hopefully make a more informed choice of food. Most flavour enhancers are commonly unnatural ingredients such as additives or include salt and increased fat levels.

DOG/CAT VERSIONS OF HUMAN FOODS, E.G. CHRISTMAS CAKE AND EASTER EGGS

More recently, there has been a rise in the popularity of humanized versions of pet foods. Pet guardians like to think they are giving their pet the best experience and so the feeding of seasonal products such as dog cake, Easter eggs, beer or Advent chocolate at Christmas is a clever marketing ploy. Pet guardians often feel guilt, when absent from their pets when at work or socializing and may choose to compensate with these types of treats. Treating a pet is not forbidden, but must be done in moderation and in consideration of the daily caloric intake in balance with exercise levels.

PET BIRTHDAY CELEBRATIONS

Celebrating a pet's birthday has become commonplace in many families. They are part of the family, after all! Pet parents will mark the occasion with toys, treats and some will even throw a party As a one-off, people tend to overlook calories and nutrient content although it is wise to consider and offer food in sensible amounts due to the richness which could cause an upset stomach. The level of fat and calories within treat foods should be compensated with adjusted amounts of the daily diet.

Trends are often followed by pet guardians and sometimes without the necessary research. It is common for people to be influenced by what they see on social media: a large following can build momentum which makes a product appear to be more credible than it actually is. The most important message is that pet guardians must carry out the necessary research on a product before making impulse purchases. Animal industry practitioners must be up to date with current trends and up to date with the latest brands and feeding methods in order to correctly advise the consumer.

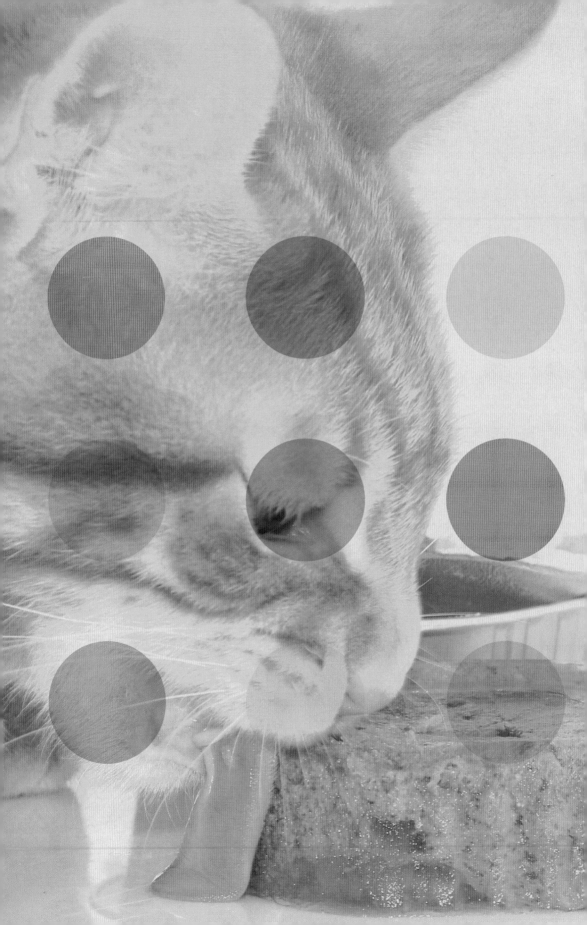

07

ASSESSMENT
OF AVAILABLE DIETS

AVAILABLE DIETS

Complete diets are by far the most convenient type of food to offer your pet since they contain the key nutrients for the species, age and life stage. This type of food is designed to be fed on its own and there is no requirement to add additional foodstuffs which would unbalance the caloric intake. Complete foods are available in wet, semi moist, dry and raw forms.

In contrast, complementary foods can be fed depending upon owner preference and should be fed with caution since the individual components (i.e. mixer) do not contain all the necessary daily nutrients that a complete food does. Some owners like to provide variety for their pets and may chose this route or a home-prepared food.

Similarly, home-prepared foods are not complete and the owner must carefully research dietary requirements for the species, breed, life stage and satiety status of the animal. This option is preferred by many who are conscientious about the traceability of ingredients and quality in terms of natural and organic food sources.

A simple and common way to bulk out complementary diets is to add a cereal-based mixer which, depending upon the quality may have additional vegetables and herbs for improved palatability and higher nutritional content. It is important to note that mixers increase the carbohydrate content of food but do not provide significant nutritional benefit and are typically included in complete foods as a cost-effective bulking agent. The low digestibility of such bulking agents lead to a higher percentage of waste matter, hence causing the dog to defecate more frequently and it can have varying amounts and consistency and a more unpleasant smell.

TYPES OF DIET

Wet food

Wet foods have a high water and meat content and while tinned, pouched and tray foods are convenient to feed, they are also relatively expensive to feed on a daily basis. Typical daily feed amounts are also high in wet foods to compensate for the high water content and reduced energy density and the cost factor is a significant consideration for pet owners.

The quality of meat in wet foods is variable and the nutrient content can vary between batches, especially when animal derivatives are listed or the food is labelled as a particular 'flavour'. When packaging is labelled as 'chicken flavour', for example,

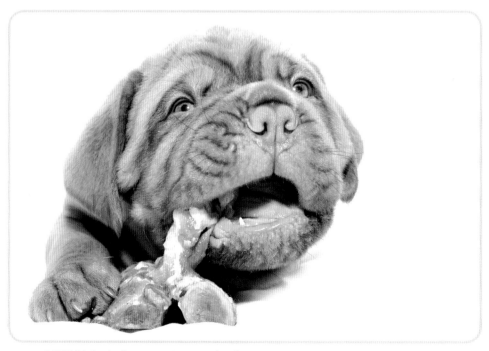

↘ BARF (biologically appropriate raw food).
Photo: Adobe Stock – jandix2

the product only has to contain a minimum of 4% chicken and the rest of the protein can be made up of any other meat source that is cost-effective at the time – hence why the nutrition can vary between batches.

The typical wide range of flavours of wet foods are a popular choice for pet guardians since humans tend to take an anthropomorphic view; it can be difficult for some people to comprehend feeding the 'same thing' every day, because 'it must be boring' for the animal. Wet foods are highly palatable and visibly pleasing to animals which is why they are rarely refused and are more appealing for owners. Moreover, wet foods can be preferred by vets when recommending diets for animals recovering from illness and in particular those with diagnosed kidney problems when an increased water content is needed.

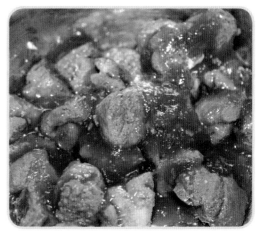

↘ Wet food.
Photo: Pixabay

Moist food is preserved appropriately and has a long use-by date but when opened can be rather unpleasant smelling and can spoil quickly, therefore it requires refrigeration.

Semi-moist food

Semi-moist food is typically packaged in trays, foils or sachets and is available in varying forms from high-quality fresh meat/fish with vegetables and/or rice. In comparison, this type of diet can also consist of meat derivatives and cereals bound together with some sort of syrup and water, cooked into a paste or soft pellets. The water content is moderate compared to a wet food but significantly higher than a dry food. As per wet foods, semi-moist foods are highly palatable

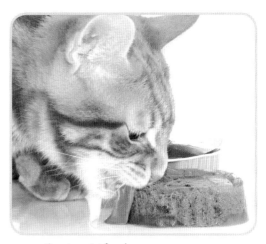

↘ Semi-moist food.
Photo: Adobe Stock – illustrez-vous

and digestible but tend to have increased salt and sugar levels. These foods have a long use-by date and once opened should be consumed within a few days but semi-moist foods do not necessarily require refrigeration due to preserving agents. The cost of these foods is wide ranging and brand-specific.

Dry food

While convenient to prepare and feed, dry dog foods are extremely variable in quality and price. It is pertinent to say that the cost of dry food is not necessarily reflective of quality and it is imperative to educate in pet food labelling to ensure safe and appropriate selection.

Unquestionably, dry foods have a very low moisture content of approximately 10%, are typically packaged in bags or boxes that have a long shelf life and require storage in a cool, dry place. Exposure to moisture will spoil the quality of the food and allow for possible contamination.

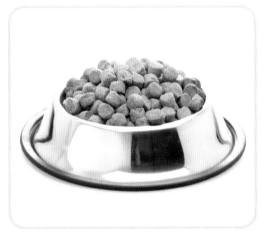

↘ Dry kibble.
Photo: Adobe Stock – BillionPhotos.com

Dry food should be fed in its natural state although some pet guardians insist on adding water (cold or warm) or gravy for their own reasons, although advice would be to refrain from this since it contradicts the nature of dry food in aiding dental health. Dry food also encourages increased water consumption, which is important to prevent dehydration and promote kidney health; therefore, fresh water must always be available.

One of the initial considerations when deciding on a dry food is whether to opt for a complete or complementary diet depending upon preference and budget. Second, it is important to read the order of ingredients on the food analysis, as previously discussed in Chapter 4. In most cases, it is preferable to select a food that lists protein as the main ingredient; this can commonly be dry meat, fresh or bone meal, and so on.

The next step is to assess the source of protein and its biological value which will have a direct impact on the nutrient density of the dry food. Ideally, it is better to find a food that contains a named meat meal source such as 'duck meat meal' so that there is higher reassurance that the end product actually contains a minimum of 20% of the specified animal. Another good source is fresh meat which is highly palatable and of good quality, although its high water content reduces the overall quality of the protein once processed. Again, the source of protein should be specified, otherwise the product lends itself to an 'open formula'. Animal derivatives are a low-grade quality protein and are typically associated with reduced cost.

Carbohydrates are a necessary food source for energy but are not the primary source of energy, therefore it is common for manufacturers to use cheap and often nondescript forms of carbohydrates in the form of 'cereals'. In this case, it is safe to assume that there are unknown sources and quantities of carbohydrate, which lends itself to an open formula. This use of cereals makes food more difficult to digest, can reduce palatability and furthermore can make food-associated allergies more difficult to identify. When open-formula cereals are used, the need for enhancing palatability is rectified by adding salts, flavours (often artificial depending upon the brand) and fats to make the food more enticing, although this can be detrimental to health.

RAW diet

Raw foodism is growing in popularity and is a popular lifestyle choice followed by owners. Food traceability is important to owners and the feeding of uncooked and unprocessed food is preferred by many, due to control over the source and quality of food given to their pet. This is otherwise difficult to do with a proprietary diet. Feeding of raw food is a relatively recent concept and is considered as a contentious topic in the field of pet nutrition because of the risk of uneducated owners providing diets with unguaranteed nutritional value and caloric content. There is also

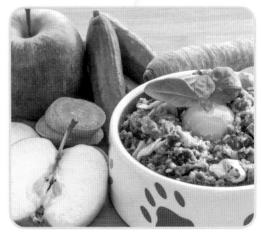

↳ Raw food.
Photo: Adobe Stock – Lilli

the risk of exposing their animals to harmful bacteria such as E. coli. Pet guardians will need to be educated or supported in raw feeding to be confident that they are supplying a safe and balanced diet.

There are companies that manufacture raw-based diets specifically balanced to meet nutritional needs of the species and breed of animal; these can be seen as a safer and more reliable choice than the owner calculating the diet themselves. Feeding RAW diets does not come without risk and possible unwanted complications, a big risk being that of E. coli and storage issues.

Care must also be taken when preparing this type of diet and strict hygiene practised:

○ Wash hands before and after preparation
○ Wipe spills immediately
○ Use separate chopping boards for preparation
○ Wash the pet's bowl immediately after eating.

Vegetarian diets

Vegetarianism is a philosophical lifestyle choice that some humans like to impose upon their pet and there are considerations that need to be carefully quantified in order to be confident that it is safe and appropriate. This is especially true in the case of felines as they are obligate carnivores and require a strict meat-only diet to ensure they receive essential taurine and arachidonic acid which cannot be synthesized from other nutrients in the body as in other species. Taurine is not present in the right quantities in dog food, hence why it is not appropriate to feed dog food to cats. Additionally, deficiencies in taurine and arachidonic acid can lead to night blindness and nutritional illnesses such as hypertrophic cardiomyopathy, therefore a meat-free diet is not suitable for cats.

Dogs are omnivores and can synthesize specific nutrients such as arachidonic acid from linoleic acid, unlike obligate carnivores. This would suggest that canines are more tolerant of a vegetarian diet or the feeding of a raw or home-made diet.
If you are considering feeding your pet a home-made RAW diet, veterinary advice is recommended for nutritional support before doing so.

Breed-specific diets

Breed-specific diets are readily available on the market, which have different kibble shapes and sizes to suit the breed and reflect breed-specific nutritional requirements.

These can be recommended by veterinarians following diagnosis or breed-related issues.

Supplementation

Many pet guardians are turning to natural ingredients to supplement a pet's diet; most of these are mainly anecdotal but have positive reports in humans. Fish oils have had noted benefits for many years and in recent years coconut oil, aloe vera and turmeric have grown in popularity with claims to aid with skin and coat condition, help with joint issues, improve digestion and improve immunity. Coconut oil is a good form of fat but if offered should only be fed in small quantities and not fed to already overweight dogs; too much can cause diarrhoea. It is important that supplements should never be used as an alternative to veterinary treatment but they can be used to complement a good-quality diet.

LIFE STAGE FEEDING IN CANINES

Animals require different levels of nutrients at different stages of their life, therefore it is important to adjust the nutrient intake according to age, breed and health status.

Puppy

Energy and nutrient levels are in much higher demand in growing animals and their diet should have a higher nutrient requirement to support development. In the first two weeks of a puppy's life, it spends much of its time sleeping and feeding but there is no need to supply additional food at this stage as the puppies rely on the mother's milk for nutrition. The weight of a healthy puppy will double in just a few days therefore close monitoring of the puppies and dam is essential during this time to ensure she is tending to the puppies and has a constant supply of milk.

Weaning will start at 3–4 weeks old with the gradual introduction of a nutritionally-balanced puppy kibble which, mixed with water, can be offered four times a day. The puppies will rely on the mother's milk initially until fully weaned at around 6–8 weeks old, by which time the mother will no longer allow suckling and the puppies will feed independently.

A balanced diet must be provided for steady growth of bones and joints as a deficiency can result in skeletal disorders such as osteochondrosis. Consideration for large and giant breeds should be key since the calcium to phosphorus ratio is different to that of medium or small breeds and imbalances at this stage can have a dramatic effect on development.

CASE STUDY

NERO

Nero was a healthy 4-month-old puppy. His pet guardian ensured that he had a monitored level of exercise and caloric intake according to the feeding instructions on his diet sheet. He had reached the age to be moved onto a junior diet programme. This was to ensure he had all the appropriate nutritional balance to encourage the next life stage (junior) and he would continue to remain fit and healthy. His owner transitioned Nero over a 14-day period to minimise any digestive upset.

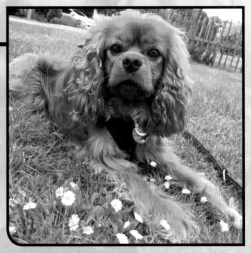

→ Nero.
Photo: Tony Keegan

Junior

A dog reaches the 'junior' stage at around 6 months old, but this depends on the breed as large or giant breeds take much longer to reach their adult size/weight.

Gestation and lactating

Reproduction is very demanding on the body, can be stressful and can drain the bitch of energy. It is not uncommon for the mother to become deficient and therefore she needs a high-protein, energy-dense diet. She will need to be offered food three to four times that of her maintenance requirement.

Food does not need to be increased until the third trimester as this is the point at which most of the foetal growth takes place. The bitch can be offered food little and often as large volumes of food cannot be tolerated at this stage of her pregnancy. During lactation, the diet needs to contain enough energy to support the production of milk, moreover it has a higher fluid requirement to promote milk supply.

Adult

A typical adult dog will be fed a good-quality, balanced diet for maintenance levels to ensure enough energy is supplied for daily activities. Additionally, energy is also important for defence of disease, good digestive function and to promote a healthy coat condition.

Senior

Generally, a dog is classed as senior at around 7 years of age but this depends on the breed. For example, a Border terrier is renowned for having a longer lifespan but in contrast a Great Dane will reach 'senior' years at approximately 5 years old since they generally have a shorter lifespan.

The transition to a geriatric diet should happen before the signs of ageing appear, as by this time the effects of old age have already taken effect. A senior dog will have less demand for energy and changes in requirements for nutrients such as protein. Protein should be provided in lower quantities compared to a typical adult food but the protein should be of a higher biological value.

CASE STUDY

JACK

Jack, a 7.5-year-old German shepherd dog lives with his elderly owner in her 70s. Unfortunately due to ill health Jack's owner was unable to provide the same level and intensity of exercise. Coupled with the natural ageing process, Jack is less active on his walks and subsequently has recently gained weight. Jack is currently still fed an adult diet which is providing more energy than he is able to burn. It has been identified that Jack needs to make the transition onto a senior food which is less calorie-dense and will see him through his senior years.

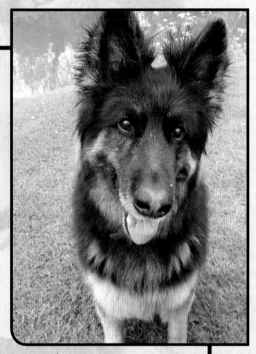

↪ Jack.
Photo: Helen Coleman

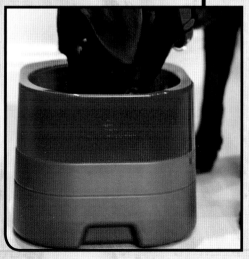

↪ Elevated feeding for geriatric pets may provide a more comfortable feeding position.
Photo: PetWeighter

Reduced protein lowers the risk of obesity and fat levels in proprietary diets should be reviewed to ensure that they are not above 10%, which is in line with a weight-controlled diet. A senior dog requires around 20% less energy than an adult dog as they are generally less active and undertake less exercise because their energy metabolism becomes reduced.

> **HANDY HINT**
>
> An example of a higher biological value protein could be salmon which is protein-dense and contains less fat.
>
> ○ ○ ○

Geriatric dogs commonly experience renal problems which impact the diet provided. Consideration of the type of protein should be made to supply a good-quality protein to reduce stress on the kidneys as a result of less waste product.

Phosphorus levels should be reduced to prevent wear on the kidneys and liver; commonly a proprietary diet will have reduced phosphorus levels.

Water-soluble vitamins such as B and C need to be increased to compensate for reduced function of the kidneys.

Working dogs
Working dogs can be classed as:

○ Racing dogs
○ Sprint racing dogs (e.g., greyhounds)
○ Endurance racing dogs (e.g., sled dogs).
○ Other working dogs, such as:
○ Military and police dogs and other dogs trained to detect explosives and drugs
○ Dogs trained to assist disabled people
○ Farm dogs
○ Dogs taking part in competitions (e.g., agility competitions).

Dietary needs of a working dog depend on the type of activity and weather conditions. Dogs that are exposed to the elements need more energy to support a healthy body condition and a change of diet may only be needed on a seasonal basis. A more energy-dense diet can be achieved through introducing higher protein and fat levels rather than additional carbohydrates which are not suitable to sustain energy requirements of a working dog. Increasing meal sizes will not compensate for the energy needs of a working dog as these dogs cannot necessarily tolerate large meals. Concurrently, an ample supply of water should be made available to aid hydration.

LIFE STAGE FEEDING IN CATS

Pregnancy and lactation

A feline guardian would treat a pregnant cat very much the same with ad libitum feeding which will allow the queen to self-regulate food intake and satisfy energy requirements. A typical adult food is sufficient until the third trimester when protein requirements are greater to ensure good health and reduced mortality in the developing young. There is a greater need for energy during the latter stages of pregnancy when the key neurological developments of the kitten occur. This is the time to transition to a high-protein diet which also contains a good source of omega-3 fatty acids.

As with most pregnant animals, queens need greater levels of calcium and phosphorus than in normal adult maintenance to support skeletal development of the foetuses.

Lactation is the most energy-demanding stage and drains the cat of nutrition, affecting the body condition and coat quality. Peak milk production typically occurs at three to four weeks of lactation and even with feeding the queen ad libitum, she will still need an energy-dense diet for milk production.

Adult cats

Adult cats should be provided with a nutritionally-balanced diet for maintenance, disease defence, good digestive function and to promote a healthy coat condition. Satiety status of the cat needs careful consideration when selecting the most appropriate diet due to the prevalence of urinary tract disorders, particularly in sedentary, middle-aged, male cats. Furthermore, sodium and phosphorus levels should be reviewed in regards to long-term kidney health and function.

Senior cats

As with all senior animals, cats generally become less active as they age which is associated with a slowing metabolism and lower satiety levels. As a result, a good-quality senior cat diet will need to be provided to supply good levels of vitamins and minerals for aiding the ageing process. A good source of protein will compensate for reduced gustation and olfaction sense, hence selecting a food with

CASE STUDY

OBI

Obi is an approximately 14-month-old rescue cat who had been placed in temporary fostering care. Once her pregnancy was detected she was then placed on a growth diet appropriate to support the latter stage of gestation. This diet has a high-protein value to support the energy demands of the growing foetuses. She delivered four kittens successfully; it is recommended at this stage to place the cat on a life stage diet to support lactation but unfortunately a charity cannot fund this type of diet. Instead, the closest alternative was to continue on a growth food to provide enough protein to meet the high metabolic demands of lactation. At the point of writing this book, Obi and the kittens are doing well.

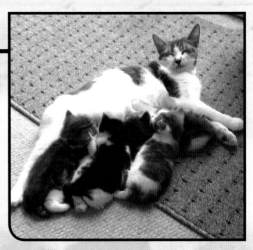

↳ Obi.
Photo: Sarah Pointer

a high biological value protein will aid palatability and increase digestibility to promote kidney function. A quality protein source fed in reduced amounts will provide sufficient energy and coupled with good-quality carbohydrates, will help to balance weight. High levels of protein, if not burnt off, will be stored as fat and create high levels of urea putting more pressure on the already ageing kidneys. An ad libitum feeding style is preferred over time-restricted to encourage the cat to feed little and often which mimics typical feeding patterns of the healthy cat, particularly geriatric ones.

FEEDING IN SUMMARY

Any pet guardian should ensure that they provide a balanced diet that contains the essential nutrients needed to provide a complete diet that meets the individual animal's needs for its life stage and physiological status.

The quality of the food fed should be taken into consideration with regards to cost, efficiency, and palatability for the animal but moreover there should be awareness of key concepts of proprietary diets to avoid clever marketing influences.

→ **ACTIVITY**
Questions:

1. Identify three key considerations of feeding for each life stage.
2. Name each of the six essential nutrients and how they should be adjusted for each life stage.
3. Compare and contrast a complementary and complete diet.

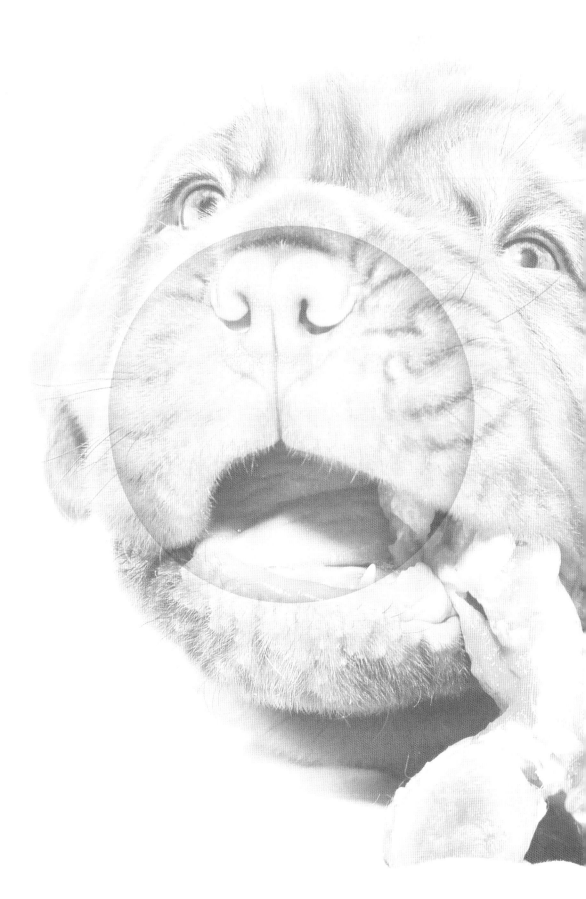

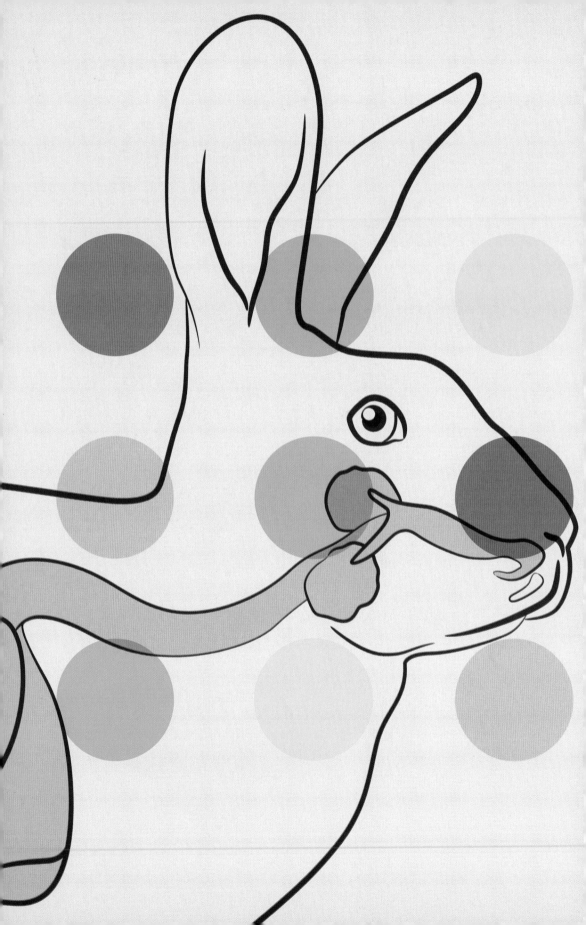

08

BASIC OVERVIEW OF
THE DIGESTIVE SYSTEM

○ ○ ○

DIGESTIVE SYSTEM

The digestive system is an important system of the animal's body. If the digestive system is upset with a disease or incorrect feeding, this can have serious implications for an animal's health. Digestive health is a must-have and all pet guardians should be advised on how to ensure this.

THE DIGESTIVE SYSTEM OF DOGS AND CATS

Let's start with the digestive system of the dog and cat.

An important part of the animal's digestion, as described in Tables 8.1 and 8.2 (overleaf), is when the deciduous (baby teeth) and adult teeth come through in dogs and cats.

○   Incisors are for picking or nibbling of food
○   Canines are for holding prey
○   Premolars and molars are for the shearing of meat.

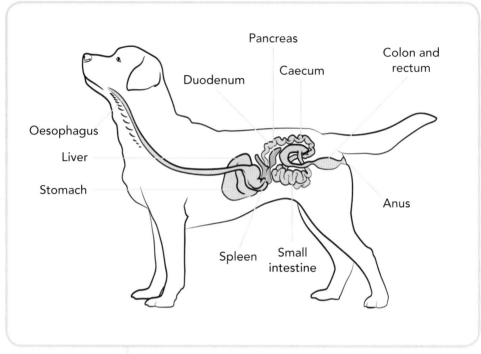

↳ Digestive system of the dog.
Artist: Jorgen McLeman

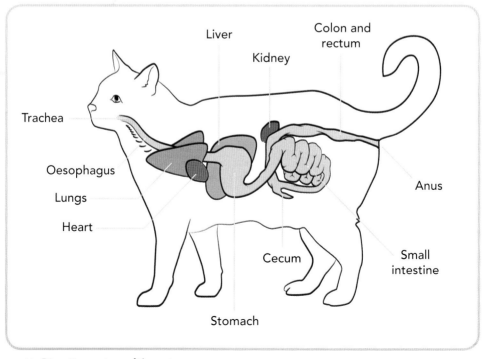

↳ Digestive system of the cat.
Artist: Jorgen McLeman

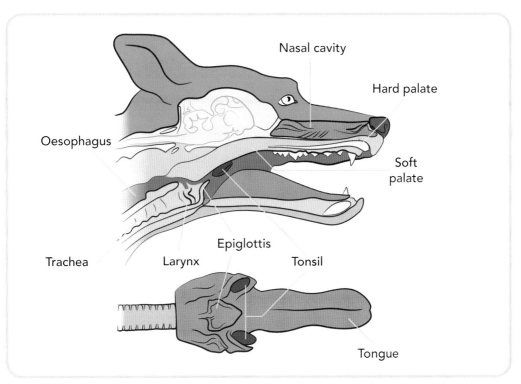

↳ Dog mouth.
Artist: Jorgen McLeman

TABLE 8.1
DECIDUOUS TEETH

TYPE	DOG	CAT
Incisors	3–4 weeks	2–4 weeks
Canines	5 weeks	2–4 weeks
Premolars	4–8 weeks	2–4 weeks
Molars	Absent	Absent

TABLE 8.2
ADULT TEETH

TYPE	DOG	CAT
Incisors	3.5–4 months	12 weeks
Canines	5–6 months	Variable By 6 months
Premolars	4–5 months (1st) 5–7 months (rest)	Variable By 6 months
Molars	5–7 months	Variable By 6 months

Dentition
- Deciduous dog: 3/3, 1/1, 3/3, 0/0 = 28
- Adult dog: 3/3, 1/1, 4/4, 2/3 = 42
- Deciduous cat: 3/3, 1/1, 3/2, 0/0 = 26
- Adult cat: m3/3, 1/1, 3/2, 1/1 = 30
- Other species' dentition:

Rodents are gnawing mammals and have sharp incisors which curve, and flat cheek teeth for chewing. Commonly, rodents' teeth are orange/yellow.

Guinea pigs and chinchillas and rabbits have creamy teeth; all teeth are open rooted although the incisors grow quicker than the cheek teeth.

Salivary glands
Saliva has a pH of about 7.8 in the dog and cat and is stimulated by various things such as the expectation of food. Saliva contains 99% water and the rest is made up of mucus. There are four pairs of salivary glands: parotid, mandibular, sublingual and zygomatic. The main function of saliva is to moisten and lubricate food. The parotid gland produces amylase in dogs which starts the digestion of carbohydrates.

Hard palate
This is a solid area which separates the buccal and nasal cavities.

Soft palate
This is a soft, fleshy partition at the back of the mouth which separates the nasal and oral pharynx; the soft palate is involved with swallowing.

Pharynx
This is the tube that connects the mouth to the oesophagus.

Oesophagus
This is the tube that connects the mouth to the stomach and uses the process of peristalsis to move the food.

Stomach
This is divided into different sections and holds the food. It is also the site for chemical and mechanical digestion. It also controls the release of the food into the small intestine.

Chyme

After a couple of hours of digestion, the stomach content is now termed chyme with a pH of 1.5–2. This is slowly released into the small intestine.

Small intestine

This is the main area of chemical digestion and absorption of the nutrients. It consists of the duodenum, jejunum and ileum.

Secretions of the small intestine include:

- Bile
- Pancreatic juice
- Intestinal juice.

Bile

The gallbladder produces bile in reaction to the presence of chyme. Bile salts emulsifies fats and activates lipase for the digestion of fats.

Pancreatic juices

- Amylase breaks down carbohydrates.
- Trypsin breaks down protein.
- Lipase breaks down fat.

Large intestine

This is made up of the caecum, colon, rectum and anal sphincter and is the place where water absorption takes place. Also, it is the site for microbial digestion of fibre.

Rectum

This is where faeces are stored prior to excretion.

Anus

This is the orifice where faecal matter is expelled.

THE DIGESTIVE SYSTEM OF BIRDS

The digestive tract of the bird is different to that of mammalian digestive systems. It is important that pet guardians understand the difference to ensure digestive health of their pet birds.

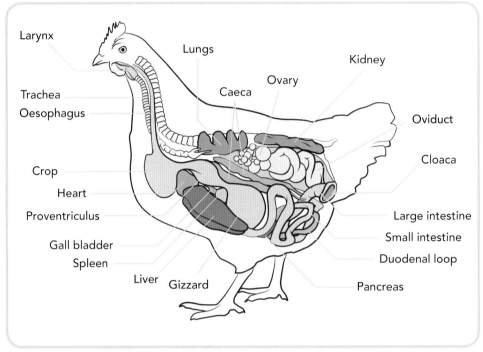

↳ The digestive system of a chicken.
Artist: Jorgen McLeman

The shape of the beak and tongue varies according to the diet and lifestyle of the species of bird. They have no teeth, but the upper beak has sharp cutting edges called tomia.

In some birds, the oesophagus has a pouch called the crop. This is used for storage; it may also produce crop milk, which is used to feed the young. The stomach consists of the:

○ Proventriculus: like the mammalian stomach, this is a glandular structure producing hydrochloric acid, mucus and pepsin
○ Gizzard: a muscular pouch used for grinding of food. Many birds ingest grit or stones to aid this process.

The small intestine is divided into the duodenum, jejunum and the ileum.

Most birds have two caeca. Digestion of bacteria takes place here. The termination of the digestive tract is also common to the urinary and genital tracts. This is called the cloaca.

The kidneys secrete solid uric acid rather than urea as in mammals. Birds do not have a bladder; therefore, water will be absorbed through the rectum.

RABBIT

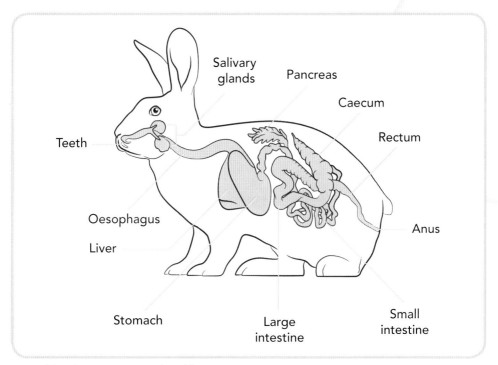

↪ The digestive system of a rabbit.
Artist: Jorgen McLeman

A key thing to remember with rabbits is that the initial digestive system is exactly the same as most mammals. The ingestion starts when the rabbit eats and the food travels from the mouth into the oesophagus. The oesophagus leads to the stomach which then goes to the small intestine. The small intestine is very important for absorbing the key nutrients from the food. Enzymatic digestion takes place, breaking down individual nutrients into an easy absorbable size; this is then absorbed into the bloodstream. Enzymes are unable to break down fibre; in most mammals, the fibre is passed as waste; in rabbits, the colon divides the fibre into two types: digestible and indigestible. The digestible fibre is passed into the caecum for processing. The indigestible fibre is essential to the digestive process for carrying food through the digestive system. This food is then passed out by the colon as hard, round droppings. During this process, a specific type of bacteria ferments the digestible fibre and breaks it down to allow the release of the stored nutrients. The caecum can absorb some of the nutrients but most need to go back into the small intestine to be absorbed. This is completed by the fermented fibre moving back to the colon where it is coated with mucus; this then is excreted as caecotropes. The rabbit, as a caecotrophic herbivore, will then ingest the mucus-like droppings so that they pass through the digestive system again. The small intestine can now absorb the nutrients.

GUINEA PIG
Guinea pigs have a similar digestive system to the rabbit with a well-developed caecum. They practise coprophagia.

TORTOISE
The internal organs of the tortoise are similar to the mammal, except that it has an external opening common to both the reproductive and excretory tract called the cloaca.

SNAKE
The organs of the digestive tract are elongated. There is a common exit for the digestive, reproductive and urinary system called the cloaca.

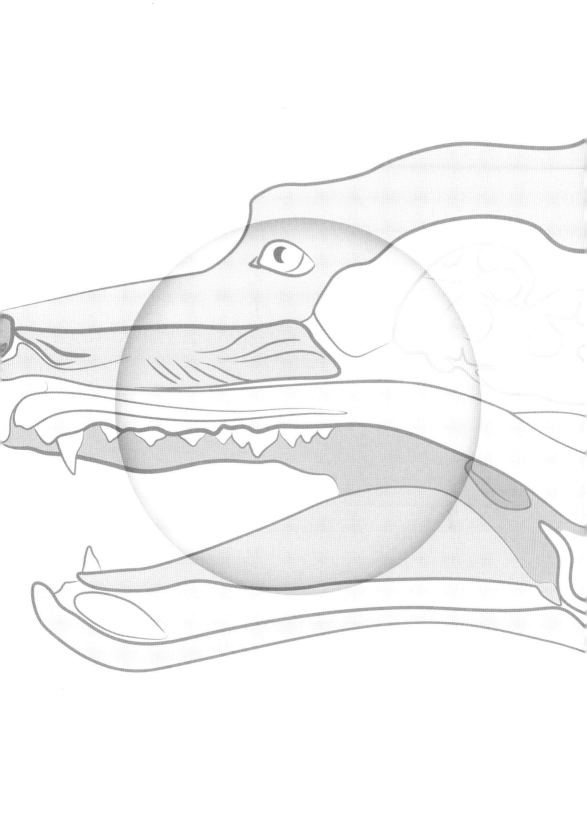

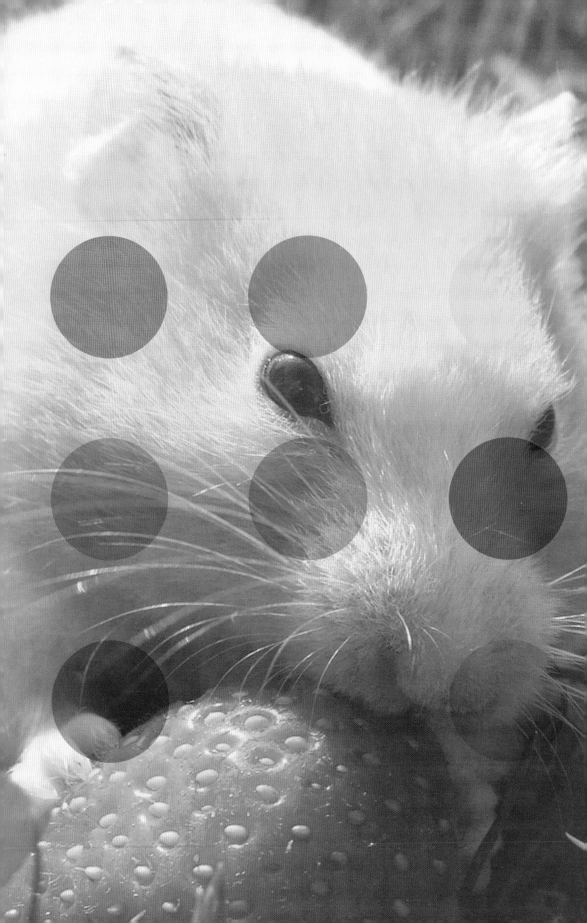

○ O ○

09
FEEDING COMMONLY KEPT SMALL COMPANION ANIMALS

○ O ○

SMALL ANIMALS ARE common pets and have daily requirements for feeding regimes. There are specific small companion animals that must have certain components and nutrients in their diet to ensure digestive health. When considering the diet of small companion animals, we must consider the following:

○ Water
○ Increase in rabbits as house pets
○ Varied diets
○ Varied nutritional and digestive set-ups
○ Amount of forms of exercise – stuck in cages/hutches.

TABLE 9.1

DIFFERENT FEEDING BEHAVIOURS WITH EXAMPLES

Omnivore: dogs, degus, rats, bearded dragons, iguanas, macaws

Herbivore: rabbits, uromastix, tortoise

Carnivore: cat, snakes, falcon, bosc monitor lizard

Group feeders: birds

Browsing: primates

Grazing: horses

Tight grazing: rabbits

Foragers: gerbil

Opportunistic: rats

RABBIT

Rabbits are foraging herbivores and spend a good proportion of their day searching for and consuming food which is naturally high in fibre. Grazing is a natural behaviour for rabbits and a diet consisting primarily of plant matter should be offered to encourage mastication which in turn wears down their open routed teeth. A rabbit's teeth have evolved to continually grow to cope with the continual gnawing and grinding.

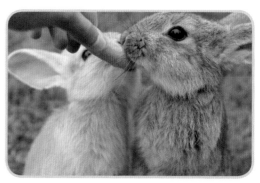

↳ Rabbits.
Photo: Pixabay

Hay and grasses should make up 80% of their primary diet which provides the high levels of fibre needed to meet natural foraging behaviours, promote good dental health and aid digestion.

Rabbits naturally have high levels of gut flora and a sudden change of diet can disrupt and disturb healthy levels of gut bacteria. Foods new to the rabbit should initially be offered in small quantities and, due to the sugar content, fruits should be offered occasionally as treat. Digestive disturbances can result in a life-threatening condition known as gustas; this requires immediate veterinary attention.

A small amount of concentrate food of approximately 25 grammes per rabbit can be offered daily as a means to supply additional nutrients and create interest. Muesli mixes are historically a popular choice to offer, however due to the likelihood of selective feeding, pelleted or extruded diets are recommended to prevent the rabbit from picking the most palatable foods over others, which can lead to an imbalance of nutrition.

A rabbit's digestive system is not designed for efficiency as they are unable to synthesize nutrients the first time food is ingested. The digestive system is functional though and although many owners do not witness reingestion, rabbits do practice coprophagia where they eat caecotrophs, a soft, brown form of faeces in order to utilise undigested nutrients. Typical faeces seen by owners and practitioners are usually the brown, hard and rounded pellets which is perfectly normal.

CASE STUDY

RUSSELL

Russell, a 6-year-old rabbit was rehomed at the age of 5. He went to the new owner with minimal medical history and has been of good health. Upon grooming, the owner noticed a swelling on his jaw and immediately sought veterinary attention. Russell was eating and drinking as normal but had become a bit more docile than normal when being groomed. The veterinary surgeon noted on inspection that he had significant molar overgrowth and his incisors did not meet naturally. This resulted in malposition and malocclusion of his hind teeth which caused sore areas on the inside of his cheeks, causing the dental abscess. Because of his age it is not recommended for him to have an anaesthetic so he was placed on palliative and symptomatic treatment until he can no longer eat or appears uncomfortable.

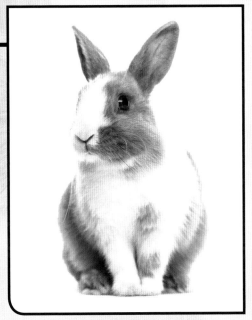

↳ Russell.
Photo: Adobe Stock – Eric Isselée

107

Failing to achieve the right balance of hay with vegetables, dark leafy greens, concentrates, treats and exercise can lead to obesity. Overweight rabbits are unable to perform the act of coprophagia and results in caecotrophs sticking to the fur around the perineum. Since the rabbit is not able to effectively clean itself it provides the ideal attraction for flies to lay their eggs, hence the onset of mydriasis, otherwise known as fly strike.

Freshly picked foods should be washed before feeding to reduce the likelihood of disease transmission from wild rabbits.

TABLE 9.2

SAFE AND UNSAFE FOODS FOR RABBITS

SAFE FOODS	UNSAFE FOODS
Broccoli	Iceberg lettuce: contains lactucarium which in large quantities is harmful to the rabbit. Lettuces that are lighter in colour contain high levels of water and therefore have lower nutritional quality.
Parsley	Legumes
Spring greens	Elder
Brussell sprouts	Deadly nightshade
Bok choy	Woody nightshade
Various herbs	Lily of the valley
Various lettuces including romaine and Boston	Lobelia
Kale can be included but must be used rarely as can be linked to bladder irritation	Foxglove
Various wild weeds – ensure they are on the safe food list	Iris
Asparagus	Ivy
Bell peppers	Yew

Note: there are many others that are safe for rabbits; this is just a small selection.

GUINEA PIG

Guinea pigs are very active diurnal rodents that can spend up to 20 hours a day foraging and grazing. Like the rabbit, they too have open routed teeth that have evolved to cope with a high-fibre diet consisting mostly of hay.

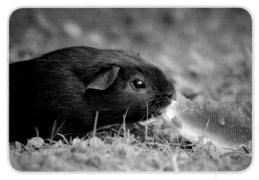

↳ Guinea pig.
Photo: Pixabay

Approximately 70% of the main diet should consist of hay and grasses along with 20 grammes of concentrates per day which is supplemented with a variety of dark leafy greens and vegetables which have high concentrations of vitamin C.

Unlike humans and primates, guinea pigs are unable to synthesize vitamin C and so plentiful amounts should be provided daily in the diet. A concentrate mix fed alone will not provide sufficient amounts and can lead to hypovitaminosis C which presents as scurvy: a painful dietary-related disease that affects the skin and joints.

TABLE 9.3

FOODS CONTAINING HIGH LEVELS
OF VITAMIN C

Kale

Broccoli

Spinach

Parsley

Bell peppers

Guinea pigs are known to practise selective feeding and therefore muesli-type foods are not recommended for this reason as the guinea pig is inclined to select its preferred foods which may not necessarily be the most nutritionally beneficial. An extruded or pelleted diet limits the opportunity to select feed and can provide some of the vitamin C requirements. Additionally, although pelleted and extruded diets often have additional vitamin C added, quantities deplete when exposed to sunlight therefore just topping up dry food is not a sufficient means of supplying vitamin C.

A vitamin C supplement can be added to water, however, guinea pigs do not tend to favour this and may be inclined not to drink as much. Furthermore, the supplement can be inactivated by the aluminium spout on a water bottle and render the supplement ineffective.

Guinea pigs practice coprophagia and eat caecotrophs which are a soft, brown form of faeces that they consume to more effectively utilize undigested nutrients. Typical faeces seen by owners and practitioners are usually the brown, hard and rounded pellets which is perfectly normal.

Failing to achieve the right balance of hay with vegetables, dark leafy greens, concentrates, treats and exercise can lead to obesity. Overweight guinea pigs are unable to perform the act of coprophagia and this results in caecotrophs sticking to the fur around the perineum.

TABLE 9.4
SAFE AND UNSAFE FOOD FOR GUINEA PIGS

SAFE FOODS	UNSAFE FOODS
Broccoli	Bluebell
Cabbage (red and green)	Crocuses
Spring greens	Daffodil
Brussell sprout	Deadly nightshade
Spinach	Woody nightshade
Various herbs	Lily of the valley
Various lettuces including romaine and Boston	Hyacinth
Kale	Foxglove
Various wild weeds – ensure they are on the safe food list	Tulip
Corn on the cob	Ragwort
Asparagus	Yew

Note: there are many others that are safe for guinea pigs; this is just a small selection.

HAMSTER

Hamsters are small, nocturnal rodents that enjoy an omnivorous diet consisting of various seeds, grains and nuts along with the occasional insect; protein should not make up more than 16% of their daily diet. A typical commercial hamster mix provides sufficient nutrition and should be supplemented with timothy hay and vegetables for additional roughage, vitamins and minerals. Fruits contain sugars and can be offered as treats for Syrian hamsters a few times a week in small amounts. Since dwarf hamsters are prone to diabetes, it is better to offer vegetables and other types of protein.

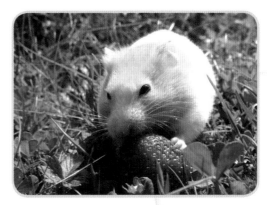

↳ Hamster.
Photo: Pixabay

Sunflower seeds and peanuts are often included in commercial mixes and although they are a good protein source, they also contain high amounts of fats and should not be offered in large quantities; fats should not make up more than 5% of the daily diet. Syrian hamsters should be offered approximately 5 grammes of commercial seed mix twice daily and dwarf hamsters a tablespoon per day. It is better to offer fresh food over manufactured treat sticks as these contain honey for binding and additional sugars which can be counterproductive to the hamster's health. Typically for rodents, the hamster's teeth grow continuously and their incisors grind together which helps to prevent overgrowth, therefore roughage helps to encourage gnawing; additionally, a gnawing block can be offered or the occasional dog biscuit.

The name hamster comes from the German word 'hamstern' meaning to 'store food' and they have pouches that start at the corner of their mouth and stretch to the shoulder blades. As hamsters will naturally stuff their pouches full of food and take it to a storage area, it is advised to offer the hamster small amounts of fresh food as it will perish if not eaten in a reasonable amount of time. Owners and animal practitioners should remove uneaten food from storage areas daily to prevent impacted/infected cheek pouches; a relatively common illness caused by the hamster putting stale food in its pouches.

Hamsters are very active animals and like wide open spaces, so providing opportunities for exercise is important in promoting their mental health through preventing boredom and keeping them at a healthy weight. As opportunistic foragers, hamsters spend a good proportion of their time searching for food, so scatter feeding can encourage activity and interest.

What foods are safe for my hamster?

TABLE 9.5

SAFE AND UNSAFE FOODS FOR HAMSTERS

SAFE FOODS FOR HAMSTERS	UNSAFE FOODS TO AVOID
Broccoli	Chocolate (contains theobromine)
Asparagus	Onion (contains theobromine)
Cabbage	Garlic (contains theobromine)
Celery	Citrus fruits
Cucumber	Dairy
Green beans	Iceberg lettuce
Corn on the cob	
Spinach	
Turnip	
Kale	
Sweet bell peppers	
Apple	
Banana	
Raisin	
Blueberry	
Melon	
Strawberry	
Occasionally	
A few pieces of hard-boiled egg – can be a useful protein addition	
A small piece of mild cheese	
Mealworms	
Cooked chicken or turkey	
Plain tofu	
A small piece of dry, plain toast	
A small dog biscuit	

RAT

Rats are omnivorous, therefore achieving a balanced diet is not difficult due to the array of different foods they can have. A commercial mix should make up approximately 80% of the staple diet and should be offered in small amounts twice daily. A nugget-type food eliminates the likelihood of selective feeding as rats are more inclined to pick out the most fatty foods when offered muesli mixes which can lead to a nutritional imbalance.

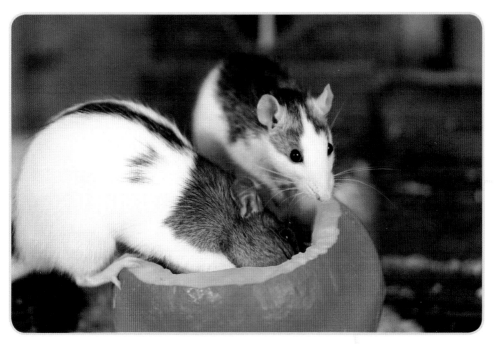

↘ Rats.
Photo: Pixabay

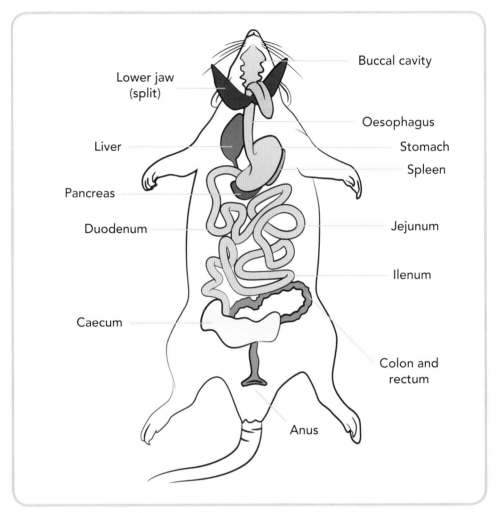

Lower jaw (split)

Liver

Pancreas

Duodenum

Caecum

Buccal cavity

Oesophagus

Stomach

Spleen

Jejunum

Ilenum

Colon and rectum

Anus

↳ Digestive system of a rat.
Artist: Jorgen McLeman

A high-fibre diet can be supplied through offering a range of fruit and vegetables; furthermore, scatter feeding creates more interest, increased activity levels and provides enrichment.

Rats are nocturnal so will consume most of their food at night and the feeding pattern should represent their activity times. It would be sensible to offer fresh food in the evening when they are most likely to consume it.

TABLE 9.6

SUITABLE FRUIT, VEGETABLES AND TREATS FOR RATS

SUITABLE FRUIT, VEGETABLES AND TREATS FOR RATS	UNSUITABLE FRUIT, VEGETABLES AND TREATS FOR RATS
Apple	Sweet potato
Cherry	Uncooked beans
Banana (not green)	Chocolate
Strawberry	Cabbage
Raisins	Brussel sprouts
Melon	Green potato
Grapes (seedless)	Onions
Blueberry	Rhubarb
Broccoli	Citrus fruits
Asparagus	
Avocado (not the skin)	
Peas	
Carrot	
Kale	
Romaine lettuce	
Celery	
Parsley	
Pumpkin	
Bok choy	
Mealworms	
Small dog biscuits	

SMALL AND VERY OCCASIONAL TREATS

Carob chip

Almonds, walnut and Brazil nut – can be given in shell

Sunflower seeds

Rice cakes

Cooked rice or pasta

A small piece of cheese, occasionally

MICE

Mice enjoy an omnivorous diet and as typical opportunistic feeders will eat most foods offered. Approximately 8–10 grammes of commercial diet should be offered in small amounts daily. Muesli mixes offer variety and interest but like other rodents, mice will also pick out the most palatable components and leave others, resulting in a nutritional imbalance. Moreover, muesli mixes are likely to contain sunflower seeds and peanuts, which are a good source of protein but also fat, and too many can lead to obesity and should therefore be limited to a treat food only. A pellet mix may appear less interesting to the human but provides reassurance that the mouse is receiving the correct nutrition.

The diet should be supplemented with small amounts of fruit and vegetables which is enriching for the mouse as they provide variety and interest. New foods should be offered in small amounts and introduced gradually. Scatter feeding small rodents encourages natural behaviours and increases activity levels which is important for mobility and reducing the likelihood of obesity. Uneaten fresh food should be removed daily to prevent bacterial growth; if the mouse was to eat the mouldy food it may cause an upset of the very fine balance of safe bacteria in the mouse intestine resulting in digestive upset.

TABLE 9.7

SAFE AND UNSAFE FOODS FOR MICE

SAFE FOODS FOR MICE	UNSAFE FOODS TO AVOID
Apple	Citrus fruits
Strawberry	Onion (contains theobromine)
Melon	Chilli pepper
Pear	Jalapeno pepper
Kiwi	Mango
Bok choy	Potato
Cucumber	Garlic (contains theobromine)
Carrot	Chocolate (contains theobromine)
Broccoli	Grapes
Romaine lettuce	Raisins
Parsley	Rhubarb
Sweet potato	Walnuts
	Iceberg lettuce

OCCASIONALLY

A small amount of peanut butter
– monitor artificial sweetener levels (xylitol)

Peanuts

Sunflower seeds

Stale wholemeal bread
(should be completely dried out then soaked in water)

Mealworm

Cooked pasta (preferably wholemeal)

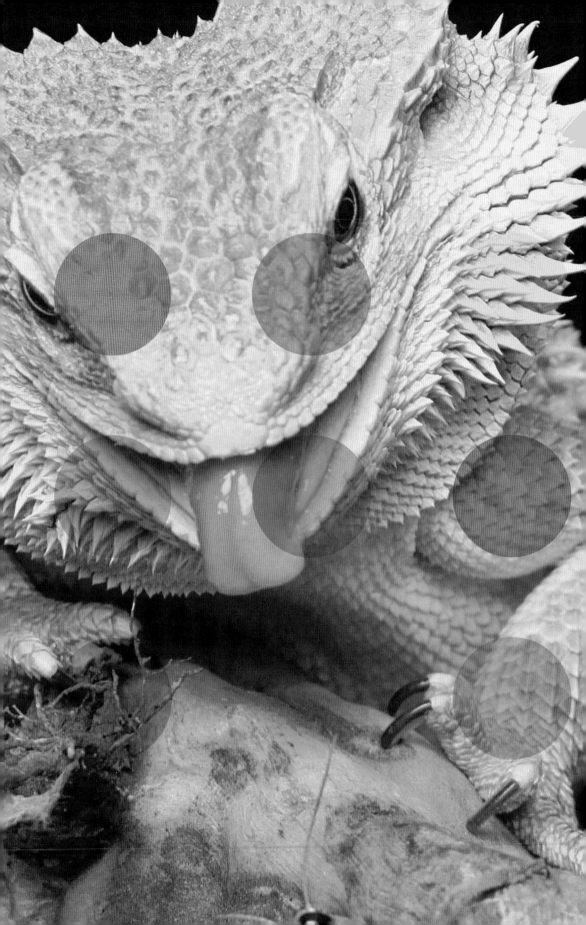

10
FEEDING COMMONLY KEPT EXOTIC PETS

EXOTIC PET OWNERSHIP is getting more popular and fashionable. Lizards are becoming one of the most purchased exotic pets in the UK. One of the main issues with exotic pets is lack of education about the species-specific care for these animals. One must ensure that, when considering one of the exotic pets, there is enough information to enable pet owners to make educated nutrition and diet choices. Many of the reptilian species need supplements and additional environmental measures to ensure they are at optimum health.

DEGU

As small caviomorphs, degus are strictly herbivorous and naturally browse on a high-fibre diet consisting of plants, leaves, bark and seeds of shrubs. Degus are adapted to a high-fibre diet and are known to practise coprophagy in order to absorb nutrients. Alfalfa hay is an excellent high-fibre, protein-based plant that offers the necessary roughage degus require as a staple part of their diet; it is difficult to break down and requires

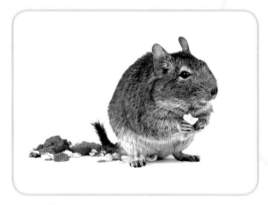

↳ Degu.
Photo: Adobe Stock – Klaus Eppele

119

chewing to wear down their continuously growing elodont teeth. There are commercial diets available specifically manufactured to meet the dietary needs of the degu which are free from molasses and low in sugar. Similarly to rodents, they too are likely to select feed and a pellet or nugget-type food will help to eliminate this practice which can lead to malnutrition. Foods for other animals should not be fed to degus due to unknown quantities of ingredients, particularly sugar ones. Sugary foods should not be fed to degus as they are very sensitive to these and it can lead to the development of diabetes mellitus. Ten grammes of dry concentrate can be offered daily to the degu and should be available ad lib due to their diurnal behavioural patterns. Additional to dry concentrate and alfalfa hay, vegetables can be offered in small quantities to enrich and provide a variety of vitamins and minerals. Small animal treats should never be offered as they contain free sugars which are intolerable and can lead to the onset of diabetes.

> **ISSUES**
>
> Susceptible to developing diabetes mellitus if fed diets with free sugars.
>
>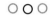

TABLE 10.1
SAFE AND UNSAFE FOODS FOR DEGUS

SAFE FOODS TO FEED A DEGU	FOODS TO AVOID
Green beans	Red and green peppers
Broccoli	Fruits
Asparagus	Small animal treats
Fresh grass	Dried herbs
Celery	Beetroot

OCCASIONALLY
Peas
Carrots
Apple
Cucumber
Sweet potato (raw and peeled)

CHINCHILLA

Chinchillas are small, crepuscular rodents that are active during twilight hours. Chinchillas naturally consume a plant-based food consisting primarily of different grasses, leaves, twigs, stems, roots, berries and bark.

Chinchillas are adapted to consume a fibre-rich diet and their open rooted teeth continually grow as a result of the fibrous diet; they should therefore be offered roughage ad lib to prevent dental disease such as malocclusion and molar route overgrowth.

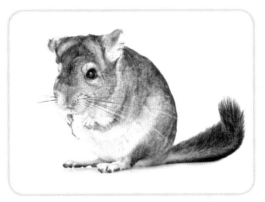

↘ Chinchilla.
Photo: Adobe Stock – Wolna

Alfalfa hay is a type of legume hay with high calcium and phosphorus levels, containing approximately 14% plant protein and closely matches desired protein levels. Timothy hay is fibrous and can also be combined, offering sufficient levels for adult chinchillas at approximately 6–8%. Plant proteins are significantly important for the formation and quality of a thick coat and digestive health.

Pellets should be available ad lib and should make up approximately 20% of the overall diet along with constant access to hay, herbs, vegetables and fruits. The occasional treat of dried fruit such as raisins may be fed as long as it does not have any additional sugars. Sunflower seeds and nuts are enjoyed but should be avoided due to the high fat content. Chinchilla pellets provide better dental protection in comparison to a cereal-based mix, which is known to encourage selective feeding and selection of the softer components which do not wear down teeth. Pellets are fortified with vitamins and minerals to ensure the chinchilla receives desired amounts.

Fresh, clean water is also important for digestive health and should be readily available to ensure the chinchilla keeps hydrated and to promote the absorption of nutrients from food.

A GENERAL GUIDE TO FEEDING REPTILES

Housing and nutrition directly correlate with the health of reptiles and there are some general principles that all reptile carers must consider to promote health and well-being.

As poikilothermic animals, reptiles have specific husbandry requirements and heat is especially important for thermoregulation, since they rely on the external temperature to regulate their body temperature. All reptiles have a preferred optimum temperature zone which is the ideal temperature essential for bodily functioning such as digestion of nutrients. Baines (2017) refers to reptiles as 'solar-powered' because ultraviolet lighting plays a significant role in the synthesis of previtamin D_3, essential for bone health. Reptiles have an effective method of filtering UV rays via the parietal (or third) eye which senses light and is able to convert UVB rays to utilize dietary calcium. Reptiles need calcium supplied within the diet to ensure that they have sufficient levels within the blood to prevent taking stores from their bones, leading to metabolic bone disease.

Although tortoises will generally shelter from the peak sun, they spend large quantities of time in direct sunlight and therefore require a calcium supplement in their diet and UVB radiation from artificial lighting in captivity. The Mediterranean tortoise is a selective browser and naturally consumes an array of different plant matter, flowers, leaves, grasses and berries. As opportunists, they may also occasionally eat the odd insect but protein should not be offered on a regular basis as tortoises are designed to digest a high-cellulose diet and proteins can lead to stress on the kidneys and eventually renal damage. Pelleted foods can be offered as an addition to plants, vegetables and salad items but not as a regular primary part of their diet as these too contain protein and levels can build to unsafe amounts and again can be linked to kidney failure. Pyramiding of the scutes can be an indication of too much protein and poor vitamin D_3 levels.

Primarily, the diet of a Mediterranean tortoise will comprise of a calcium-rich, high-fibre diet to ensure good digestive health. Cuttlebone can be left in the enclosure as an additional source of calcium of which the tortoise may consume small amounts occasionally; furthermore it is recommended that food is dusted or coated with a calcium powder two to three times a week. Too little fibre in the diet can lead to gastrointestinal upset.

Providing a diet that promotes natural grazing behaviours provides interest for the tortoise and stimulates natural feeding behaviours. Allowing the tortoise to graze encourages activity and therefore is good for maintaining weight; the Jackson ratio is an accurate way to measure weight against the length of the tortoise to learn the ideal weight for the tortoise.

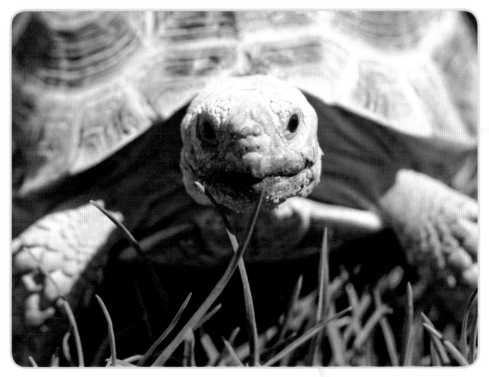

↳ Tortoise.
Photo: Adobe Stock – nagydodo

TABLE 10.2

SAFE AND UNSAFE FOOD FOR TORTOISES

SAFE FOODS	UNSAFE FOODS
Rocket	Cabbage
Lambs lettuce	Spinach
Romaine lettuce	Chard
Basil leaves	Bok choy (or any related vegetable
Parsley	as these inhibit calcium)
Prickly pear cactus (Opuntia) pads and	Parsnip
flowers (excellent source of fibre and has	Onions
good calcium–phosphorus ratio)	Root vegetables (high in digestible
Dandelion	carbohydrates)
Grass	Peas and beans (high in protein)
Barley	Kale
Cat grass	Broccoli
Timothy hay	
Honeysuckle	
Bramble	
Clover (red and white)	
Petunia leaves and flowers	
African violet	
Chickweeds	
Roses: leaves and petals	
Hawkweeds	
Hibiscus leaves and flowers	
Evening primrose leaves and flowers	
Geranium flowers	
Plantains	
Cat's ears	
Wild clematis	
Garden mint	
Oregano	
Spider plant	
(can be used to decorate the enclosure too)	

OCCASIONAL FOODS

Fruit (high in sugars and can cause gout)
Apple
Banana
Blueberry
Cress
Cucumber
Thyme

FEEDING TERRAPINS

Terrapins can have a life expectancy of 30 years in capitivity. There has been an increase in the number of chelonia species being kept as pets: this could be because of the popularity of the TV show *Teenage Mutant Ninja Turtles*. Any chelonian species can carry salmonella, which is zoonotic. Zoonoses is the spread of infection from animal species to man. There is a 90% chance that terrapins can carry *Salmonella enterica* (Ward, 2000).

Red-eared slider (Chrysemys scripta elegans)

These are extremely popular kept pets in the US. They are semi–aquatic, seen basking on rocks and logs above water level and will spend most of their time in or around water. Red-eared sliders will need a naturalistic environment that mimics their natural habitat which includes full–spectrum UV lighting and a temperature of 75–86°C for thermoregulation.

Maintenance of the water is important to promote health since terrapins will eat in the water (absence of mucus glands) and food debris will contaminate the water. A good filtration system will aid in promoting a good water quality and prevent the need for daily cleaning. The removal of uneaten food can also help prevent any build-up of waste products.

They are classified as opportunistic feeders which means they will eat anything that they come across in their natural environment. They are quite messy feeders and it is extremely important that waste food is removed and disposed of correctly.

Young red-eared sliders are carnivorous and can have a daily diet made up of crickets, mealworms, pinkies, whitebait, mussels, tubiflex worms and blood worm.

Adults can eat this fresh food less often: approximately 2–4 times a week is recommended. It is key that this does not make up more than 25% of their total diet as this can cause dietary deficiency. Adults are omnivores and plant vegetation should make up 50% of their diet; this could be in the form of apples, grapes, bananas, dark leafy greens and tomatoes.

Fresh food should be dusted twice a week with a retivit powder to ensure sufficient amounts of nutrient are digested; this is to ensure good bone health and avoid issues such as metabolic bone disease. Gut loading, as previously discussed in this book, can be used to provide the additional supplements along with UV lighting. Cuttlebone can also be provided as a supplement. Pre-pelleted food can be offered as an alternative, but it must not be more than 25% of the diet (Kaplan, 2014).

LEOPARD GECKO

Leopard geckos are nocturnal animals that have specially adapted colour vision and the ability to dilate their pupils very wide in order to locate prey in the dark. Leopard geckos will eat a varied diet of insects and arthropods that are highly nutritious and replicates the type of diet they could consume in the wild. When feeding in captivity, it is important to use a reputable supplier which will go some way to assuring the quality of the insects fed to the geckos. The owner or practitioner can take

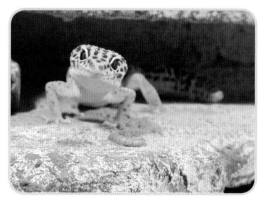

↳ Leopard gecko.
Photo: Adobe Stock – fotos4u

additional steps to 'gut load' the insects and feed them on a diet of bran along with a small offering of fruit, vegetables or salad items. Bug gel is an effective way to keep insects hydrated but they will gain moisture from food offered; furthermore, care of insects prior to feeding preserves the quality of prey to provide optimal nutrition. Geckos will be offered insects two to three times a week and it is commonplace to 'dust' or coat insects with a vitamin and mineral powder twice a week. It is important to be mindful not to 'over supplement' due to the possibility of excess fat-soluble vitamins causing toxicity. Feeding live food to geckos is not only a natural form of feeding to stimulate natural predatory behaviours but encourages activity to locate and consume the insect. That said, it is advised not to leave live insects in the vivarium for long periods as they are known to nip the gecko. A gecko may not take food each time it is offered, so keeping regular feeding and weight records is one way to monitor a gecko's feeding patterns and prevent over- or under-feeding.

Crickets are a standard, staple part of a gecko's diet and offer a lean protein. Insects offered should not be more than half the length of the gecko's head.

Mealworms are a good protein source and can be offered as an alternative to crickets but not necessarily as the staple diet due to their poor calcium to phosphorus ratio.

Locusts offer a good protein source and are generally sweeter compared to a cricket, and waxworm can be a tasty treat although should only be offered occasionally due to the high fat content.

BEARDED DRAGON

Bearded dragons are omnivorous animals and protein should make up approximately 75% of their diet which can include insects such as crickets (cost-effective and readily available), mealworms, waxworms (occasionally as they are very sweet), locusts (lean protein) or even small vertebrate animals such as (the occasional) pinkie. Gut loading of insects is important to ensure that they are of good quality and nutritious for the animal being fed.

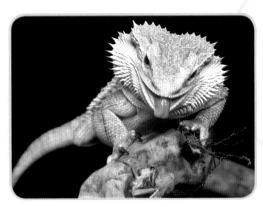

↳ Bearded dragon.
Photo: Adobe Stock – Mirko Raatz

Feeding live invertebrate animals promotes natural feeding behaviours and leads to increased activity to catch the prey. Obesity is becoming more common in captive bearded dragons due to limited opportunities for exercise and overfeeding. Too much protein in the diet can lead to renal failure, therefore it should be offered several times a week as opposed to daily. It is suggested that the amount of live food eaten is monitored and excess insects are removed from the vivarium. For example, it is known for crickets to nibble the bearded dragon when they are resting, which can later lead to small bite wounds with the possibility of developing infection. It might be suggested to remove the bearded dragon from its enclosure and feed in a separate, small, plastic vivarium to aid monitoring. Growing and juvenile bearded dragons should be given supplements more regularly while growing to promote healthy bones and joints.

It is recommended that 25% of the diet should consist of vegetables, salad items and some fruit. A variety of foods should be given (see Table 10.3) as too little variety can limit nutrition. Commercial pellet diets are available and offer a balance of nutrition; these can be sprinkled onto fresh food but are not a preferred substitute for fresh and live feeds.

Food should be dusted with calcium powder and alternated with a multivitamin powder twice a week to ensure the diet is sufficiently supplemented. Restrictions in calcium and an imbalance of phosphorus can lead to metabolic bone disease which is avoidable with correct husbandry (balance of heat and light). Over supplementation of vitamins and minerals can lead to toxicity, the quantity and frequency should be monitored. Live feed can be placed into a small plastic container with the calcium powder and given a gentle shake to fully coat the insect.

TABLE 10.3

SAFE AND UNSAFE FOOD FOR LEOPARD GECKO

SAFE FOOD – VEG/FRUIT MUST BE PEELED AND CUT INTO TINY PIECES	UNSAFE FOOD
Crickets	Iceberg lettuce
Mealworms	Spinach – contains calcium
Kingworms	absorbers which can lead to MBD
Waxworms	Avocado
Earthworms	Rhubarb
Cockroach	Fish
Locust	Seafood
Kale	
Parsley	
Clover	
Broccoli	
Courgette	
Kiwi	
Melon	
Sweet potato	
Mustard greens	
Dates	
Mango	
Bell pepper	
OCCASIONALLY	
Sprout	
Tomato	
Blueberries	
Banana	
Grated carrot	
Grapes	
Cucumber	

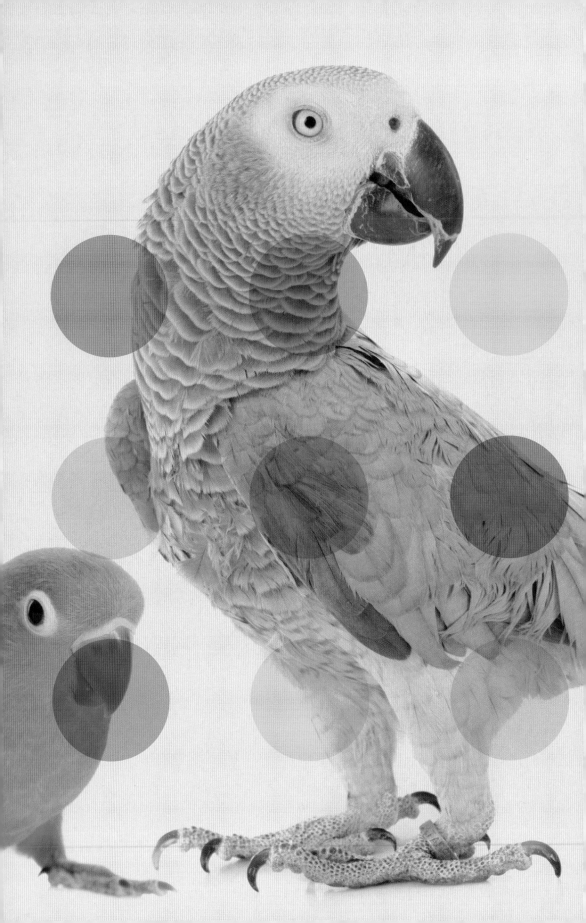

11

FEEDING COMMONLY KEPT PET BIRDS

○ ○ ○

BIRDS HAVE BEEN the pet of choice for many since 1504 (Scott, 2015). Popular for their colourful plumage, birds are very intelligent and inquisitive in nature. Many have the ability to mimic, which makes them an interesting companion for as many as one million owners in the UK (PFMA, 2015). Parrots and parakeets alike make excellent companions, forming strong social bonds, but taking on a pet of this calibre requires time and commitment. Smaller parakeets such as budgies and cockatiels can live for approximately 12–15 years, however, psittacines such as the Meyer's parrot and Hahn's macaw could exceed 30 years of age. One of the most recognisable parrots, the African grey, could live above 60 years, moreover the blue-and-gold macaw could live well into its 70s. In the UK, the pet guardian or practitioner has the responsibility under the Animal Welfare Act 2006 to provide mentally and physically for these animals, supplying appropriate housing and enrichment, sociability, veterinary care and correct nutritional support.

Siebert and Sung (2010) document 9000 living bird species with over half making up the order Passeriformes. Passeriformes, commonly referred to as perching birds, also include Columbiformes (pigeon family) and Galliformes (chicken-like birds (Veterinary Practice Publishing Company, 1996)) although most passerines maintained as pets include finches and canaries (Nijboer, 2015a; Siebert and Sung, 2010).

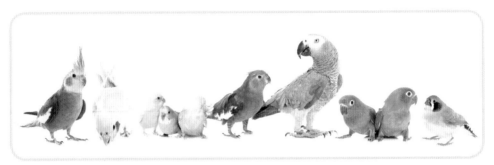

↘ Various kept bird species.
Photo: Adobe Stock –cynoclub

Moreover, most pet birds are from the Psittaciformes parrot family (Nijboer, 2015b) and include 268 species of parrots (parrots, macaws, conures, rosellas, parrotlets, parakeets, lovebirds, budgerigars), 55 species of lories (lories, lorikeets), and 19 species of cockatoos (cockatoos, cockatiels (Veterinary Practice Publishing Company, 1996)). Those kept as pets are commonly considered seed eaters, but studies of these birds in the wild have revealed that their natural foods are very different from the commercial seed mixtures typically offered in captivity (Orosz, 2013).

Most pet retail outlets will sell a traditional seed mix consisting of buckwheat, canary grass seed, corn grain, hemp seed, millet seed, oat groats (dehulled oats), peanuts (with or without shell), pepper pods and seed, pumpkin/squash seed, rapeseed, safflower seed, sunflower seed and wheat. The seed mix for psittacines will additionally contain peanuts, pine nuts, monkey nuts, dried fruit and dried chillies.

A complete food is essential to promote optimum health, and to achieve a balanced diet supplements will need to be offered.

It is important to replicate the natural diet of the bird in captivity as closely as possible and therefore a commercial seed diet is usually the obvious choice. The range of seeds offered in these diets go some way to provide a good range of nutrients, however, these have been criticized, as the main food source in the wild has not coevolved with their food supply in captivity. Furthermore, the nutrient content of a seed mixture may be very different from what is consumed (Orosz, 2013), as seed choices of captive birds are often inappropriate. Many birds are inclined to practice selective feeding and pick out their preferred food items such as sunflower seeds and peanuts. Needless to say, high amounts of fat in seed-based diets can lead to obesity and to nutritional disorders (Nijboer, 2015b).

CASE STUDY

CHOP

Alternatively, home-made diets or 'chop', as it is referred to, is a mixture of fresh and cooked foods cut very finely (or you can blend very lightly in a food processor) so the bird is unable to pick out its favourite pieces; it is particularly good therefore for fussy eaters or introducing new foods. Birds will need to be weaned onto this type of diet if they are not already familiar to get them used to the different texture. Preparation does not have to be laborious: you can make it in batches, freeze and use when required. This way, it is just as convenient as opening a bag of dry seed mix.

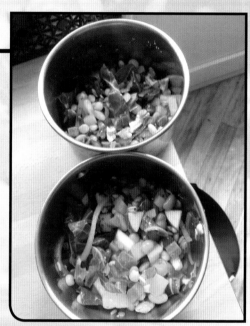

↳ Chop.

Photo: Reb Davis

Unfortunately, many commercial diets are typically low in calcium and will not reflect seasonal variances that would exist in the wild. The danger of food preference can lead to nutritional deficiencies, obesity, liver disease and gastro intestinal infections. It can also be a primary cause of feather plucking, poor feathering, and beak overgrowth and flaking (SGV Vets, 2014).

TABLE 11.1
SAFE AND UNSAFE FOOD

SAFE FOODS	TOXIC FOODS
Sweet potato	Chocolate
Carrot (roots and tops)	Onion
Salad cress	Avocado
Parsley	Fruit pits
Broccoli	Caffeine
Green beans	Mushroom
Squash	Uncooked beans
Sugar snap peas	Rhubarb
Spinach	
Red, yellow and green peppers	OTHER FOODS – COOKED
Cucumber	Pasta
Apple (seeds removed)	Wholegrain brown rice
Grapes	Quinoa
Mango	Egg in small quantities
Kiwi	Small amounts of poultry and other cooked meats
Pineapple	
Peaches	
Grapefruit	
Pears	
Oranges	

In their native habitat, birds will spend large amounts of time foraging for food and in the process will select a range of plant matter (fruits, buds, shoots, seeds, corns), and omnivorous species such as cockatoos and macaws will also ingest invertebrates.

The majority of seeds offered in commercial diets are hulled; these are a source of fibre, vitamins and minerals but are easily husked and discarded, hence the content of the food may be very different to that consumed by the bird. Moreover, husked seeds are generally lower in calcium, somewhat higher in protein, and much higher in phosphorus and fat (Veterinary Practice Publishing Company, 1996). This can lead to imbalance if activity levels in captivity are comparably lower than in the wild.

A solely seed-based diet is not a sufficient means of providing a balanced diet and feeding this alone will inevitably lead to some form of dietary-related disorder as fat-soluble vitamins A, D_3, E, and K are generally low. Deficiencies in protein, calcium and vitamin A are common, the latter more prolific in the African grey.

On the other hand, excessive amounts of vitamins can be equally as concerning and can lead to toxicity, so must be offered with care. Vitamin A deficiency has historically been noted in psittacines on all-seed based diets, so a vitamin and mineral supplement is commonly recommended (Nijboer, 2015b). Vitamin D plays an important role in the absorption of calcium and phosphorus and is generally found in low quantities when fed a solely seed-based diet. Vitamin D can only be acquired through the diet or direct sunlight, therefore the incidence of Vitamin D deficiency in captive birds is more likely due to limited exposure to sunlight, as they are often housed entirely indoors (Nijboer, 2015b).

In captivity, the large majority of birds require grit to aid digestion and this is especially true for passerines who crack open the seed hulls, whereas this is not essential for psittacines who are able to dehull seeds before ingesting. Pigeons and doves, on the other hand, must have grit available constantly as they swallow seeds whole and grit is therefore essential to promote good digestion.

There is much debate as to whether captive birds fed on a good-quality commercial diet need grit as the seeds are easily digested; the jury is still out on this dilemma. In the meantime, it is thought to be good practice to regularly supplement to ensure that the necessary resources are available for birds to choose. There are commercially available traditional grit mixtures which look very much like fine gravel, are insoluble and cannot therefore be digested. There is some concern of potential impaction if the bird consumes too much of this type of grit since it sits in the gizzard and cannot be passed through the digestive system. Furthermore, soluble forms of grit are available and can be given in the form of oyster shell or cuttlebone. Both forms are digestible and dissolve, thus avoiding impaction as they can be easily digested by the bird.

If fed an improper diet, birds can suffer from nutritional disorders, and iodine deficiency, causing goitre, is one of many and known to especially affect budgerigars. Iodine affects the function of the thyroid gland and deficiencies of this mineral cause the gland to enlarge which can impede hormone production and cause the body to produce higher hormone levels. That said, overfeeding iodine can cause toxicity which can in turn lead to overstimulation of hormone production, resulting in the enlargement of the thyroid gland. Since a commercial seed diet cannot necessarily guarantee vitamin and mineral levels, iodine should be offered regularly to ensure the bird is given the opportunity to consume sufficient levels.

Obesity in birds can be defined as the bird being 20% over the ideal weight with a body condition score of 4 or 5 (Hoppes, 2015) and, given the opportunity, birds will often select seeds with a higher fat or protein content (see page 8).

Flight requires a colossal amount of energy, so birds have developed a super-fast metabolism because of this, hence the need for food to be available ad-lib to sustain energy demands. This could go some way to understanding why birds tend to favour higher-fat seeds, however if the prevalence of fatty seeds consumed is larger than the energy expelled then the likelihood of obesity increases. Diets can be rationed in a controlled quantity but less than the animal's desired ad lib intake (Zuidhof et al., 1995; Danielsen & Vestergaard, 2001; de Jong et al., 2005; cited by D'Eath et al., 2008) to manage the weight of the bird. Food can be reduced in quality and still offered ad lib, but this is termed qualitative restriction (Sandilands et al., 2005). Such diets are an effective means of food restriction because ad lib-fed animals consume less energy from low-quality foods (Brouns et al., 1995; Savory et al., 1996; West & York, 1998; Whittemore et al., 2002; Tolkamp et al., 2005; Johnston et al., 2006; cited by Phillips, 2016).

When replenishing food bowls, it is relatively common practice to dispose the remainder of seeds from the food pot each day and replace with fresh seed. Owners and animal practitioners are advised to be vigilant when replenishing seeds to monitor food consumption so it can be noticed if the practice of selective feeding is evident as it is likely that the same seeds are left untouched each day. A more economical way of replenishing food and to encourage the bird to consume a wider range of seeds would be to give the food pot a gentle shake so that the empty seed husks will rise to the top. The empty seed hulls can then be removed and only a necessary amount of seed topped up.

Pelleted and extruded diets have tremendously improved the nutritional intake and subsequent health of captive birds (Nijboer, 2015a). It is considered a more reliable way of offering a complete and balanced diet with a guaranteed nutritional balance, omega-3 fatty acids as well as probiotics (Nijboer, 2015a) to ensure required levels are met (Veterinary Practice Publishing Company, 1996).

Despite nutritional benefits, a pelleted diet can be criticized for its lack of forage-like opportunities (Rozeka, et al., 2010) as less time is spent on food selection and manipulation which reduces activity and naturalistic behaviours. Diets offered in captivity are energy-dense and while they may provide to a degree some foraging opportunities, they take much less time to consume than other foodstuffs such as fruit and vegetables. Supplementing with fresh food is an additional novel method of adding variety, interest and more of a challenge, which promotes mental stimulation. Most importantly, fresh fruit and vegetables when fed alongside a pellet or seed diet are an additional source of vitamins and minerals. Moreover, they take longer to consume which utilizes more of the bird's energy and uses their time constructively. Scatter feeding is a good way to mimic natural foraging behaviours for small passerines (Siebert and Sung, 2010) but creative methods of food presentation is encouraged for all birds to increase activity of positive behaviours and promote an enriching environment.

Enrichment is an important part of avian physical and mental health. An easy way to stimulate the environment of the bird is to present food in novel ways. Van Zeeland et al. (2013) consider foraging enrichment as the most effective strategy to improve welfare, reduce stereotypies and other abnormal or undesirable repetitive behaviours. Most passerines and psittacines would naturally spend many hours a day foraging and travel to multiple food sites but the captive situation is often different. As captive birds do not necessarily have the opportunity to visit multiple food sites and this limits the energy demands that would be comparable when in the wild.

Providing the opportunity to forage in their captive environment would create a more challenging and stimulating environment. Highly concentrated diets in captivity reduce time spent feeding. Once food is consumed the animal will likely redirect their behaviour which can become destructive or repetitive such as perch hopping or feather plucking. Giving the bird plenty of opportunities to express natural behaviour will encourage good mental health.

Additionally, psittacines species in particular are very dexterous and food manipulation plays an important role in food selection. They have a tactile bill which assists them in the identification, selection and manipulation of food (Veterinary Practice Publishing Company, 1996).

Parrots are known to contrafreeload and will work for food even when food is freely available. Birds in captivity often have reduced opportunities to perform these innate behaviours and may spend as little as an hour on feeding (Oviatt and Millam, 1997; Rozeka et al., 2010; cited by Van Zeeland et al., 2013).

Food location, selection and manipulation are important behaviours associated with avian feeding and the majority of psittacines are prehensile-footed. The outer digits of the foot are rotated to manipulate the food item, this act of Podo-mandibulation is particularly strong with larger psittacines (Rozeka et al., 2010) who will lift food directly from the bowl with their foot which simply acts as a positioning tool, straight into the mouth. Other avian species, including some parrots, lower their heads to the food source itself (Smith, 1971, 1972; Harris, 1989; cited by Rozeka et al., 2010), furthermore, Amazon parrots are arboreal feeders and regularly use their beak and feet to manipulate the large food items they are accustomed to consuming (Rozeka et al., 2010).

Limiting the opportunity for avian species to carry out innate feeding behaviours can have serious consequence and result in boredom, and such frustrations are often re-directed as repetitive behaviours that have no specific function. These are known as stereotypies. Through boredom, birds are known to resort to repetitively chewing on wire bars, tongue playing, feather pecking, feather plucking or pterotillomania and other, feather damaging behaviour (Meehan et al., 2003, 2004; Lumeij and Hommers, 2008; cited by Van Zeeland et al., 2013).

HAND REARING

Birds should ideally be parent-reared to receive health-promoting intestinal flora from the parent through regurgitation. There are times when hand rearing the hatchling is necessary; feeding should not be started immediately as the chick needs time to fully consume the remaining yolk sac it was feeding on inside the egg. Feeding can commence at around 6 to 12 hours old following the first elimination of waste. The youngster should initially be fed every two hours reducing to every 4-5 hours as the chick grows. The liquid formula can be offered via a syringe, crop-feeder, pipette or even a bent spoon to form a funnel. It is important to maintain strict hygiene when hand rearing, as baby birds have limited immunity to prevent issues such as sour crop.

Weigh each baby bird first thing in the morning when their crop is empty. It is important to weigh the bird daily and record this information to know when to start the weaning process. Baby birds will be fluffy and chubby but they have to lose this weight in order to be able to fledge (fly) so they will start to feed less once they have reached their optimum weight. Naturally, the bird will drop the frequency of its feeds and will begin to lose weight; it can lose from 10–25% of its body weight but any more than this may indicate veterinary treatment is needed. At 4–6 weeks old the bird may start to play with the food as if it is losing interest and start to show an interest in solid foods and peck at seeds. At this point, offer plenty of seeds that the bird shows an interest in as well as those it ignores. Aim to get the bird used to a variety of foods such as legumes, seed sprouts and, a particular favourite for many, fresh corn on the cob. Small pieces of fruit and vegetables can also be offered for variety. Water should always be available when weaning.

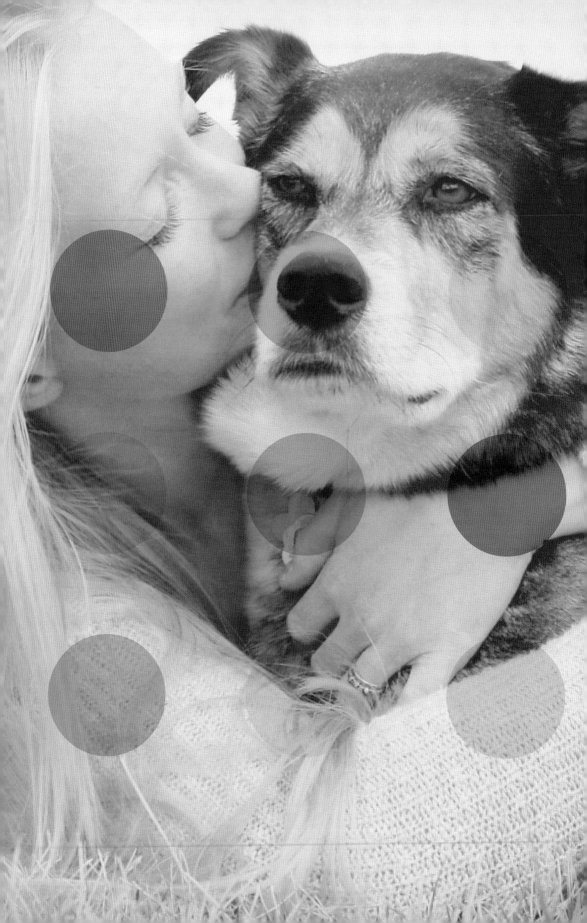

12
CONCLUSION

PROVIDING A SUITABLE DIET for your pet is a big responsibility and nutritional value is a concept that many owners do not pay enough attention to beyond fancy packaging and clever advertising. Owners often naively purchase a proprietary diet believing it is suitable but are unable to effectively assess the quality. Many cannot interpret a pet food label and pet food manufacturers are not forthcoming in making ingredients transparent.

It is the responsibility of the pet owner to effectively research suitable diets and this book is certainly a useful tool to better equip pet owners, practitioners and veterinary professionals. It is important that veterinary professionals are knowledgeable in this area because they are a source of support for owners who are unsure of the best decision for their pet. More proficient checking and recording of weight is necessary to ensure that veterinary professionals and owners can note when there has been a weight change. Early intervention can help to prevent obesity-related health issues such as osteoarthritis or diabetes; obesity is both preventable and easily treated but not through diet alone.

Owners need to honestly assess whether their lifestyle accommodates a pet, since a careful balance of exercise and diet is the most effective method of maintaining weight and diet-related health. Unfortunately, circumstances change which can often not be predicted, but a pet's diet and exercise regime also needs to adjust accordingly. There also needs to be better education with regards to body condition scoring and this is a practice that owners should be assessing regularly as second nature. It is also important that owners feel that they can go to a veterinary professional without judgement, receive productive advice and be willing to accept change. Their beloved pet may have to receive less treats; the pet is likely to appreciate attention and exercise much more than a treat which is short lived and is forgotten about in seconds. The human–pet dynamic plays a significant role in how humans see and treat their pets but food should never be a replacement for exercise or attention. A short training session, extra walk around the block, a run in the park or play with toys can help to build the human–animal bond to create a better relationship that both parties will benefit from. Obesity is a welfare issue and owners need to recognize that it is not acceptable to have an overweight pet and that obesity will compromise both the quality of life and longevity.

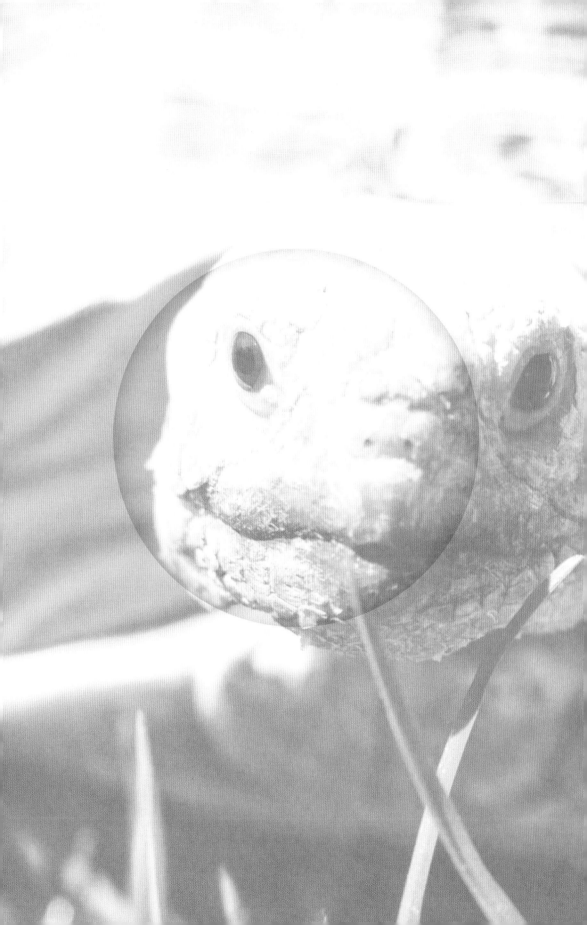

BIBLIOGRAPHY

Baines, F. (2017) [online] Captiveandfieldherpetology.com. Available at: https://captiveandfieldherpetology.com/wp-content/uploads/2017/02/Bearded-Dragon-Care-2017-Frances-Baines-MRCVS.pdf (accessed 12 March 2017).

Bland, I.M., Guthrie-Jones, A., Taylor, R.D., and Hill, J. (2008) Canine Obesity: Owner attitudes and behaviour. *Preventative Veterinary Medicine* 92 (4): 333–340.

Bren, L. (2001) Pet Food: The Lowdown on Labels (online). Available from www.fda.gov/fdac/features/2001/301_pet.html (accessed 23rd March 2014).

Cardinali, R., et al. (2008) Connection between body condition score, chemical characteristics of body and reproductive traits of rabbit does. *Livestock Science* 116: 209–215.

Courcier, E., O'Higgins, R., Mellor, D., and Yam, P. (2010) Prevalence and risk factors for feline obesity in a first opinion practice in Glasgow, Scotland. *Journal of Feline Medicine and Surgery* 12(10): 746–753.

D'Eath, R., Tolkam, B., Kyriazakis, I., and Lawrence, A. (2008) 'Freedom from hunger' and preventing obesity: the animal welfare implications of reducing food quantity or quality. *Animal Behaviour* 77: 275–288.

De Godoy, M., Kerr, K., and Fahey, G. (2013) Alternative Dietary Fiber Sources in Companion Animal Nutrition, 5 (8) MDPI (online). Available from www.ncbi.nlm.nih.gov/pmc/articles/PMC3775244/ (accessed 21st December 2015).

Dog Nutrition (2014) Dog Obesity Warning: Overweight Dogs Die Young (online). Available from www.dognutritionguide.co.uk/dog-obesity/#dog-obesity-map (accessed 23rd March 2014).

FEDIAF (2015) Legislation – FEDIAF. [online] Fediaf.org. Available from: http://www.fediaf.org/self-regulation/legislation.html (accessed 18th January 2015).

German, A. (2006) The growing problem of obesity in dogs and cats. *Journal of Nutrition* 136 (online). Available from http://jn.nutrition.org/content/136/7/1940S.short (accessed 23rd March 2014).

Harcourt-Brown, F. (2002) *Textbook of Rabbit Medicine*. Oxford, Butterworth-Heinemann.

Harvey, A. and Taylor, S. (2012) *Caring for an Overweight Cat*. Roslin, Vet Professionals.

Hoppes, S. (2015) Nutritional Diseases of Pet Birds (online). Available from www.merckvetmanual.com/mvm/exotic_and_laboratory_animals/pet_birds/nutritional_diseases_of_pet_birds.html (accessed 30th December 2015).

Kaplan, M. (2014) Red-eared Sliders (online). Available from www.anapsid.org/reslider.html (accessed 18th June 2017).

Kienzle, E., Bergler, R., and Mandernach, A. (1998) A comparison of the feeding behavior and the human–animal relationship in owners of normal and obese dogs. *The Journal of Nutrition*, 128, (online). Available from http://nutrition.highwire.org/content/128/12/2779S.short (accessed 23rd March 2014).

Lund, E. M., et al. (2005) Prevalence and risk factors for obesity in adult cats from private US veterinary practices. *International Journal of Applied Research in Veterinary Medicine* 3: 88–95.

Lund, E. M., et al. (2006) Prevalence and risk factors for obesity in adult dogs from private US veterinary practices. *International Journal of Applied Research in Veterinary Medicine* 4: 177–186.

McNicholas, J. (2005) Pet ownership and human health: a brief review of evidence and issues. *British Medical Journal* 331 (online). Available from www.bmj.com/content/331/7527/1252?ehom#alternate (accessed 23rd March 2014).

Meredith, A. (2012) Is obesity in pet rabbits a problem? *The Veterinary Record* 171 (online). Available from http://veterinaryrecord.bmj.com/search?fulltext=is+obesity+a+problem+in+rabbits+&submit=yes&x=0&y=0 (accessed 23rd March 2014).

Mintel (2011) Pet Food and Supplies (online). Available from http://store.mintel.com/pet-food-and-supplies-uk-march-2011?cookie_test=true (accessed 24th March 2014).

Mohan-Gibbons, H. and Norton, T. (2010) Turtles, Tortoises and Terrapins, in Tynes, V. (Ed.) *Behaviour of Exotic Pets*. Oxford, Wiley-Blackwell, pp. 34.

National Institute of Health (America) (2011) Overweight and Obesity Statistics (online). Available from www.niddk.nih.gov/health-information/health-statistics/Pages/overweight-obesity-statistics.aspx (accessed 14th April 2017).

Nijboer, J. (2015a) Nutrition in Passerines (online). Available from www.merckvetmanual.com/mvm/management_and_nutrition/nutrition_exotic_and_zoo_animals/nutrition_in_passerines.html (accessed 22nd July 2015). Kenilworth, USA.

Nijboer, J. (2015b) Nutrition in Psittacines (online). Available from www.merckvetmanual.com/mvm/management_and_nutrition/nutrition_exotic_and_zoo_animals/nutrition_in_psittacines.html (accessed 22nd July 2015). Kenilworth, USA.

O'Malley, B. (n.d.) Reptiles: husbandry and common conditions. *Irish Veterinary Journal* 60 (5) (online). Available from http://www.veterinaryirelandjournal.com/Links/PDFs/CE-Small/CESA_May_07.pdf (accessed 15th July 2013).

Opazo, J.C., Soto-Gamboa, M., and Bozinovic, F. (2004) Blood glucose concentration in caviomorph rodents. *Comparative Biochemistry and Physiology Part A: Molecular & Integrative Physiology* 137(1): 57–64.

Orosz, S. (2013) Critical care nutrition for exotic animals. *Journal of Exotic Pet Medicine* 22(2): 163–177.

PDSA (2014) PDSA Reveals Pet Obesity Map of the UK and Urges Owners to Take the 'Weight Off' Their Portly Pets (online). Available from www.pdsa.org.uk/about-us/media-pr-centre/news/801_pdsa-reveals-pet-obesity-map-of-the-uk-and-urges-owners-to-take-the-'weight-off'-their-portly-pets (accessed 23rd March 2014).

Pet Food Manufacturers Association (PFMA) (2015) Birds (online). Available from www.pfma.org.uk/birds/ (accessed 4th August 2015).

Phillips, C.J.C. (Ed.) (2016) *Nutrition and the Welfare of Farm Animals.* Switzerland, Springer International Publishing.

Phillips-Donaldson, D. (2012) The Latest Research on Petfood Palatability (online). Available from www.petfoodindustry.com/articles/3124-the-latest-research-on-petfood-palatability (accessed 9th January 2016).

PIF (2015). About Us. [online] Petcare.org.uk. Available at: http://www.petcare.org.uk/index.php/about-us (accessed 12th January 2015).

Raffan, A. (2014). The big problem: battling companion animal obesity. *Veterinary Record* 287–291.

Roura, E., Baldwin, N., and Klasing, K. (2013) The avian taste system: potential implications in poultry nutrition (online). Available from *Animal Feed Science and Technology* 180: 1–9 (accessed 10th December 2015).

Rozeka, J., Danner, L., Stucky, B., and Millama, J. (2010) Over-sized pellets naturalize foraging time of captive orange-winged Amazon parrots (Amazona amazonica). *Applied Animal Behaviour Science* 125: 80–87.

Rubinstein, J. and Lightfoot, T. (2012) Feather loss and feather destructive behavior in pet birds. *Journal of Exotic Pet Medicine* 21(3): 219–234.

Sandilands, V., Tolkamp, BJ., and Kyriazakis, I. (2005) Behaviour of food restricted broilers during rearing and lay—effects of an alternative feeding method. *Physiol. Behav.* 85: 115–123.

Sandoe, P., Palmer, C., Corr, S., Astrup, A., Bjørnvad, CR. (2014) Canine and feline obesity: a One Health perspective. *Veterinary Record* 175: 610–616.

Scott (2015). Pet Parrots | A Complete Beginners Guide. [online] Theparrotsocietyuk.org. Available at: http://www.theparrotsocietyuk.org/pet-parrots/a-complete-beginners-guide (accessed 10th December 2015).

SGV Vets (2014) Avian Nutrition – The Latest Recommendations (online). Available from www.svg-vets.com/avian-small-exotics/ (accessed 24th July 2015).

Siebert, L., and Sung, W. (2010) *Behavior of Exotic Pets*. Chichester, Wiley-Blackwell.

Surai, P. (2002) Natural Antioxidants in Avian Nutrition and Reproduction (online). Available from www.feedfood.co.uk/download/Imm_my_2002a.pdf (accessed 22nd July 2015). Nottingham, Nottingham University Press.

Ullrey, D., Allen, M., and Bayer, D. (1991) Nutrition of Caged Birds (online). Available from http://flightedbirds.org/fbwiki/images/1/12/Ullrey_allen_baer.pdf (accessed 1st January 2016).

van Zeeland, Y., Schoemaker, N., Ravesteijn, M. (2013) Efficacy of foraging enrichments to increase foraging time in grey parrots (Psittacus erithacus erithacus). *Applied Animal Behaviour Science* 149: 87–102.

Veterinary Practice Publishing Company (1996) Nutrition of Psittacines, Parrot Family (online). Available from www.scenicbirdfood.com/pdf/NutritionPsittacines-1009.pdf (accessed 22nd July 2015).

Ward, L. (2000) Salmonella perils of pet reptiles (online). Available from http://home. insightbb.com/~rlcc/SalmonellaTurtles.pdf. *Communicable Disease and Public Health* (3), 1 (accessed 18th June 2017).

Wedderburn, P. (2015) If Your Pet is Fat You're Now Normal (online). Available from www. telegraph.co.uk/journalists/pete-wedderburn/11504764/Why-have-our-pets-become-so-fat.html (accessed 14th April 2017).

World Health Organisation (2014) Obesity (online). Available from http://www.who.int/ topics/obesity/en/ (accessed 23rd March 2014).

INDEX

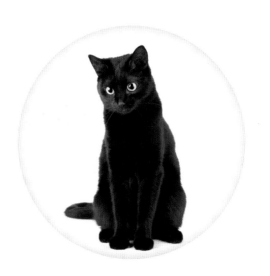